SHE'LL NEVER DO ANYTHING DEAR

A HUMAN HORIZONS SPECIAL

SHE'LL NEVER DO ANYTHING, DEAR

by

Joan Hebden

A CONDOR BOOK
SOUVENIR PRESS (E & A) LTD

First published 1985 by Souvenir Press (Educational & Academic) Ltd,
43 Great Russell Street, London WC1B 3PA
and simultaneously in Canada

ISBN 0 285 65015 7 (casebound)
ISBN 0 285 65010 6 (paperback)

Typeset by Inforum Ltd, Portsmouth
Printed in Great Britain by
Photobooks (Bristol) Ltd.

You need a sign. What better one could I give than to make this little one whole and new? I could do it; but I will not. I am the Lord and not a conjuror.

I gave this mite a gift I denied to all of you — eternal innocence. To you she looks imperfect — but to me she is flawless, like the bud that dies unopened or the fledgling that falls from the nest to be devoured by the ants. She will never offend me, as all of you have done. She will never pervert or destroy the work of my Father's hands. She is necessary to you. She will evoke the kindness that will keep you human. Her infirmity will prompt you to gratitude for your own good fortune. More!

She will remind you every day that I am who I am, that my ways are not yours, and that the smallest dust mote whirled in darkest space does not fall out of my hand. I have chosen you. You have not chosen me. This little one is my sign to you. Treasure her . . .

from *The Clowns of God* by Morris West,
Hodder & Stoughton, 1981.
Reprinted by permission of the publishers.

Contents

My intention was to record the names of all those we would like to thank for their part in helping Cathy to achieve her true potential. But the list became too long and I was haunted by the story of the Fairy at the Christening; perhaps by casting my net widely I might, by mischance, leave out one important name.

It is better, therefore, to make the list anonymous and to include:

> Our fellow members of Southend MENCAP and MENCAP National Society.
> The Down's Children's Association.
> The Staff at Lancaster School and Maybrook ATC.
> All who have been involved at any stage in the Duke of Edinburgh's Award Scheme.
> Those in guiding or youth work for the handicapped.
> A host of friendly shop assistants, bus crews and others who have helped and encouraged.
> The stars of stage, screen and air, who have given us their time.
> Our friends, who have offered support and love.

To all of these we offer heartfelt thanks and the assurance that the part they have played was a most important one.

There are some to whom I would have liked to refer by name in the text, but they are wise enough to appreciate why I have not done so. It is that kind of understanding which has made them such invaluable friends.

J.H.

Introduction

by Maggie Emslie, Director, Down's Children's Association

I would be delighted to introduce any book whose climax was the central subject's success in winning the Duke of Edinburgh Gold Award. How many of us, after all, could fulfil half the tasks demanded for completion of this prestigious achievement? I know I couldn't! Yet Cathy Hebden has done so, and Cathy has Down's Syndrome. To pay tribute to her, therefore, gives me exceptional pleasure.

Voluntary organisations such as ours strive endlessly to raise funds for expensive advertising campaigns costing tens, sometimes hundreds of thousands of pounds; Cathy's achievement, with the worldwide media coverage that accompanied it, was worth ten advertising campaigns, for in showing that she could compete on the same terms as any other young person, she has brought consolation, inspiration and hope to parents of Down's Syndrome children of all ages, to families with Down's Syndrome members and to professionals working with them. Moreover, members of the public who have never known a person with Down's Syndrome have been touched by Cathy's story and impressed by her determination.

This book, however, tells the story of a whole family, as is only right, for had Cathy's family believed the pessimistic, ill-informed medical predictions they were given in the early days, one cannot help but wonder whether Cathy would be meeting the Duke of Edinburgh this year under such auspicious circumstances.

Some readers may say that Cathy has obviously always been exceptional, and that they could not hope to achieve so much with their own Down's Syndrome child. Reading Joan Hebden's remarkable story, however, leaves little doubt that she herself is an exceptionally determined person with a very supportive family. While such qualities are important in rearing any child with special needs, we have to remember how different from today was the situation in the medical world when Cathy was born, where children like her were concerned. The term 'Down's Syndrome' was then unknown and, indeed, has only been used with increasing regularity since 1982, when the Down's Children's Association launched a determined campaign to eliminate the use of the word 'mongolism' to describe the condition, and to dispel the prejudices and misconceptions that accompany it.

Cathy, therefore, was born a 'mongol', although not immediately diagnosed as such. Today, thankfully, diagnosis at birth is usual and, with increased information about the true potential of Down's children coming from professionals and parents, combined with practical support from such voluntary agencies as the Down's Children's Association and MENCAP, such horrors as Joan Hebden describes should not occur. Occasionally and sadly, however, they still do; we have a long way to go before high-achieving young people with Down's Syndrome, like Cathy, will cease to be regarded as 'freaks' or 'one-offs'. Nevertheless, Down's babies born today enter a world of increased awareness deriving from achievements such as Cathy's, from friendships made in integrated educational settings, Brownie and Scouts packs and other leisure organisations. Even the most handicapped Down's Syndrome children are no longer hidden away and institutionalised; in general, the media seem to have opened their hearts to mentally handicapped people, perhaps reacting against the general ignorance of society until now.

There was no such emerging awareness when Cathy came into the world. In 1961, despite the high incidence of Down's Syndrome (one in 660 live births, and perhaps as many as one in 200 conceptions), these children were sadly still regarded as 'mongoloid idiots', a term unfortunately coined by Dr John Langdon Down in 1866 when he first identified the group of symptoms and called the syndrome 'Mongolism', in view of the victims' physical resemblance to people of mongol race. It was, indeed, generally accepted at that time that such children would achieve little or nothing; it was thought to be not worth spending time on them, and often not even worth taking them home. Institutions bulged with highly dependent Down's Syndrome people – dependent because they had never been given the opportunity to learn self-help skills, let alone to read, write and lead the fulfilling lives we know are possible for many Down's Syndrome individuals.

Organisations made up of parents are all too often regarded as overoptimistic, even evangelical, with an 'every home should have one' attitude, but in this book Joan Hebden is honest about the problems she has faced. Many were born from intransigence and prejudice in others, but she is careful to point out these difficulties, which any parent of a Down's child may have to face, even under the best circumstances. She is also frank enough to describe her own periodic feelings of self-doubt when working with Cathy towards another goal, and the criticisms by others of the methods she used.

In talking to parents, one of the most common questions to arise is that of just how far they should 'push' their child, whether their expectations are too high. Onlookers many sometimes be horrified, accusing them of cruelty and lack of feeling, but such reactions often stem from low expectations and even pity. These are two sentiments for which Joan Hebden had little time.

Support for Joan was not always available; professionals were sceptical and resources were poor. Fortunately we have moved far since then, but we still have far to go. While the range of professional services available to pre-school Down's children in some parts of the country is admirable, other areas are 'deserts of support' where families have to travel long distances for infrequent therapeutic appointments, and the child is forced to enter the only available playgroup, regardless of its suitability.

Attitudes are changing, but we must not be complacent. The recent uproar in the north-east, when one family wanted to open their home to five young people with Down's Syndrome, indicates the level of prejudice still prevailing in the minds of the ill-informed. Thankfully, local support won the day and that particular hostel is now open.

I firmly maintain, however, that the most effective way of dispelling prejudice about Down's Syndrome is to get to know a person with the handicap. For those readers who will never have the pleasure of meeting Cathy Hebden, this books fills that gap. Through it, we come to know Cathy and her family, and to look with understanding and admiration at the goals they have achieved. We also look forward, with anticipation, to Cathy's future achievements, and to those of the thousands of Down's Syndrome people who will accompany and follow her.

London
April, 1985

Chapter 1

Someone was gripping the small of my back with red hot pincers and churning around somewhere inside me with an exploratory knife. At least, that's what it felt like.

I tried to arrange myself into the recommended position for practising natural childbirth, but it was virtually impossible to relax and at the same time grasp the edges of the narrow couch to keep myself from falling off.

Another wave of pain broke over me like a relentless tide bulldozing its way across a placid shore. What on earth was I doing here, lying on this fiendish torture-couch, instead of in my own newly-decorated bedroom with the white-frilled cot beside me, ready to receive the newest occupant?

My mind was a hotch-potch of conflicting emotions: outrage, at having to suffer various indignities practically in public; bewilderment, because things seemed to be out of my control and happening far too quickly for comfort; intense anxiety, because at any moment my baby was going to be born and there was no one at hand to help me. I had tried to pray, but somehow the words were meaningless. Perhaps God did care, but he seemed unreal and so far away. This feeling of isolation only added to my discomfort.

Across the corridor from me, another luckless expectant mother was also battling alone. We were not able to communicate verbally but, since both our doors were wide open, we were fully conscious of each other and I felt we had a kind of kinship, in that our efforts had become a free spectacle for any interested passers-by (and many of these there were: students, clerks, orderlies and — for all we knew — even the traditional 'painter passing out for a pint'.)

The occupant of the third room was out of sight, although

definitely not out of earshot. She kept up a continuous high-pitched screaming, interspersed with a stream of profanities. I wondered how she managed to find enough breath to shriek, swear, suffer contractions and work towards producing a baby without pause — or so it seemed.

My sympathies went out to her. She must be having a very bad time; although certainly she had the benefit of the entire staff around her bed — Sister, two nurses and a medical student. As it happened, we learned later that her supposed labour had been a false alarm and she did not have her baby until three or four days afterwards. She was suffering from a neurosis which forced her to demand attention and she had put up such a great performance that everyone was fooled into believing her.

I could not help feeling that it was surely unnecessary for *four* people to dance attendance on her, even if they were convinced, because of the demoniac screams, that an emergency was about to develop. The answer that I, personally, had received, when I had at last managed to attract a nurse's attention as she passed my door, was an abortive one.

'Nurse — I really *am* well into the second stage of labour,' I had insisted desperately.

'Nonsense! You'd be making much more fuss if you were!' With a merry laugh and a friendly wave of her hand, she whisked away without coming anywhere near me.

I debated her answer with astonishment. I had been reared in a family with certain traditions of stoicism. When in pain one did not shriek or whine, but gritted one's teeth and tried to grin, however lopsidedly. To cry when you were hurt would have been considered very *infra dig*. What on earth would they have thought of me if I had bawled my head off because of the natural pangs of childbirth?

In any case, as far as I was concerned, the very strong contractions I was now experiencing would have been quite easy to bear if I had been blessed with a little human company.

The hardest part was the ever-growing feeling of terror that my baby would be born precipitously and would fall from the high, narrow couch before I could recover enough to prevent it. Surely a new-born infant would die, having crashed from a height onto a tiled floor? And the delivery couch must be at least four feet off the ground, as I had had to climb up several steps to mount it.

To my intense relief, Sister suddenly decided that our noisy fellow-sufferer should be introduced to the gas-and-air machine. The apparatus was in my room and, for some unknown reason, she came to fetch it herself. I made a last, desperate appeal.

'Sister, this baby is going to be born at any minute —'

She regarded me coldly.

'Really, you mothers . . . I never heard such rubbish!'

'Sister — please! Surely it won't hurt just to look?' The last few words came out in a strangled gasp as I felt the baby's head crown.

'Don't put on an act, now. There's no need to be dramatic,' she began, then evidently thought better of it, gave a deep and resigned sigh and moved at a leisurely pace over to my side. She lifted the voluminous hospital gown, gave an uninterested look, then I saw her facial expression change ludicrously. She called urgently:

'Nurse! The trolley — quickly!'

But she was much too late. I delivered my baby into her reluctant hands and all became confusion. I was conscious of running feet, the crackling of starched skirts around my couch, voices that said strange, unintelligible things . . .

I wallowed for a moment or two in a sense of blessed relief. By now, the baby had been whisked away and placed on the newly-arrived trolley. Everyone was crowding around it, abandoning me once again.

'Is it a boy or a girl?' I murmured dreamily, but no one answered.

They might have told me, I though resentfully, and then wondered vaguely why the baby was not crying. My other three children had all fought their way into the world yelling lustily. I became conscious of a stir of disquiet.

'Is the baby all right?' I croaked. No answer. I repeated the question with more urgency. This time Sister turned and looked at me.

'See to the mother, Nurse.'

I knew that there was more to come. The nurse, a slight Malayan girl, began to pummel my tummy. I wished she would stop.

'Nurse, is the baby —?'

'Hush, now; just relax.'

'But is it all right? Will he — she —?'

'It's a little girl.'

At this moment, a delicate thread of sound echoed thinly through the room. The baby was crying . . .

Ten minutes later, order had been more or less restored. Sister and the student had returned to their shrieking patient, who was stridently demanding their attention. The senior of the two nurses went to visit my silent neighbour, presumably to make sure that she, too, was not giving birth unattended. My little Malayan nurse began to push the baby-trolley towards the door.

'Nurse!' She halted and turned back, throwing me a shy smile.

'I will come back to you.'

'Yes, of course, but — can't I see my baby? Please?'

She looked somewhat disconcerted.

'Later, when she has been washed.'

'Oh, *please*. I *must* see her.'

She cast a nervous look in the direction of the corridor, where Sister could be heard declaiming: 'Just relax, please. Now, breathe deeply —'

Nurse scooped up the baby in one graceful gesture and held her high in the air for me to see. My daughter wailed lustily.

'Couldn't I just touch her — hold her for a minute?'

'No, no!' She hastily replaced the yelling bundle and shot out of the door.

I lay on my uncomfortable couch, unwashed and alone,

fighting off the waves of deep depression that threatened to engulf me. This should have been a moment of intense joy; anyone who has seen the radiance on the face of a newly-delivered mother will know what I mean.

How different had been the births of my first three children. Then, attended by my doctor and midwife — both old friends of the family — I had taken the whole thing in my stride. I am not going to suggest that having a baby is any picnic, but my earlier experiences had been pretty close to it.

Encouraged warmly, supported with love, there was even time between contractions for a joke or two; occasionally we had dissolved into such hilarity that I had gasped: 'Don't make me laugh any more — I can't push!'

Immediately after the birth, I had cradled each baby in my welcoming arms, studying with wonder and delight the minute perfection of fingernails like pink shells and the ridiculous toes. An immediate bond had been welded between my baby and me.

Now, I felt cheated, full of an empty frustration. The ironic part was that I had been ordered into hospital so that I might be kept under strict supervision, in case anything should go wrong.

Everything had been ready and waiting at home; Tuxie, my midwife, booked — and everyone raring to go. But my doctor had gone on holiday. She had taken off quite happily, knowing that the baby was not due for some weeks yet.

Unfortunately, my blood pressure decided to shoot sky-high and I developed toxaemia. The locum I consulted insisted vehemently that I must be hospitalised. It was to be for only a few days, perhaps a week at most, I was assured.

I hated the thought of leaving home. The hospital was quite a journey away and, in any case, they did not allow children to visit. How could I bear the thought of not seeing our three for a whole week? They were all at such interesting stages in their development. And how would they manage without me? The two elder ones were sensible enough to understand why I must go, but what about Michael? He was only four years old and would probably think I had deserted him.

All the same, I realised I ought not to take any chances. It was obvious that I *did* need complete bed-rest for a while, and it was virtually impossible to manage that at home, with a young family to look after. Maybe, just for a week . . .

Once inside, however, it became a different story. Nobody was willing to sign my release, everyone agreed it was imperative that I should stay. As the weeks went by I began to despair of ever seeing my home again.

It was decided finally that on no account must I be allowed to have a home confinement. There were all kinds of dangers attached to my condition: risk of haemorrhage, kidney failure, even eclamptic fits.

That was what made the whole situation so ironic. Far from being rigidly supervised, with every possible aid standing ready in case of emergency, I had virtually given birth all on my own! At least at home I should have been attended lovingly by friends — and highly qualified and efficient ones at that.

Now, lying waiting for someone to come and do something about me — surely they could at least give me a wash? — I compared the contrasting atmospheres of the two wards I had occupied. There was a friendly, free-and-easy air about Ante-Natal, which by no means diminished its efficiency. Sister was a darling and nurses and patients alike adored her. She was a frail-looking little thing (although actually with an iron constitution!), very feminine and attractive, and she charged to and from the hospital on an enormous motorbike. We used to see her tearing through the grounds at an outrageous speed.

She often came in to chat with us when going off duty and would sit on our beds and natter in a most un-Sisterly way. She always tried to arrange her patients into compatible groups. Thus, the four of us who occupied the glassed-in balcony at the end of the ward — commonly known as the Goldfish Bowl, for obvious reasons — were all 'hospital' types. That is, three of us had husbands in the medical world or had worked in that line ourselves, and the fourth was a trained nurse.

We were all on salt-free diets, too, and together suffered the deprivation of having to eat things like salads, steamed fish and

boiled potatoes, all utterly devoid of salt. Imagine our joy when
a student nurse, new to the ward, served us all with bacon and
fried eggs for breakfast! We wolfed it down with guilty haste,
before anyone should come along and whip it away. Although
we were all fully aware that such delicacies were definitely *not*
included in our diets, we found temptation just too hard to
resist! Actually, it did not seem to do any of us any harm
physically, but it raised our morale no end!

The same nurse — poor girl, she was always in hot water —
created another unforgettable memory for me. The weather
had turned extremely hot. We, in the Goldfish Bowl, suffered
more than anyone else in our glass prison.

Stoically we sweltered away in our thick hospital nighties,
and our delight knew no bounds when the new nurse wheeled in
a trolley loaded with clean linen. Beside the coarse, regulation
white gowns was a small pile of garments of decidedly superior
quality. They were made of soft lawn-like material and almost
transparent. Unfortunately, we found that there were only
three of them; we tossed up and I lost. The others gloated away
happily, lying tauntingly on top of the bedcovers in their
diaphanous white nighties.

I had the last laugh, though. Sister came in all too soon and
stood for a moment, dumbfounded.

'Holy Saints!' she finally exclaimed. 'What in the name of
God are you all doing wearing shrouds?'

Yes, we certainly had our moments of fun in Ante-Natal. It
was no wonder that someone once said the archway leading to
the Labour Ward should bear the notice, 'Abandon hope, all ye
who enter here'. The ward had a very bad reputation and all
kinds of stories had leaked back to us, of patients having their
babies on trolleys in the corridor, while waiting for a bed, or
sustaining bad perineal tearing because of lack of attention at
the moment of birth.

I had taken all these horror-stories at face-value, knowing
how quickly rumours can spread. Now, I was beginning to
believe them all.

It seemed to me that from the moment I entered the Labour

Ward I had contrived to antagonise Sister. She had adamantly refused to let me make a 'phone-call to Donald, my husband, to let him know that the baby was on the way. Quite apart from the fact that I had rung him daily from Ante-Natal, I felt that he had every right to know what was happening, since it was his baby, too!

I had put my foot in it, too, by being what she termed 'bossy' and trying to tell her how to do her job. Actually, I had felt it only fair to warn her that my last baby had been born after only two hours of labour. It was quite conceivable that the same thing might happen again, so I had been told. Having reprimanded me, she cast one last withering glance in my direction and then left me severely alone — except for one brief visit some time after lunch had been served.

The hospital food varied considerably from day to day, according to which chef was on duty. One of them was a superb cook and turned out delicious dishes, most attractively garnished; the other executed (good word!) some atrocious recipes, presumably using the same ingredients as chef A, but managing to get incredibly weird results. (A typical example was popularly known as 'Kit-e-Kat Pie'. Heaven alone knows what it actually contained, but the contents really *did* look and smell exactly like that well-known catfood!)

Today's offering — by chef B, needless to say — was boiled mutton. It had been left on my locker during my absence in the examination-room and was already completely cold. Grey lumps of unappetising and very fatty meat swam in a sea of grease. I was beginning to feel very queasy and had to turn my head away to prevent myself from retching. I certainly could not bring myself to tackle it, and pushed my locker a few inches further away so that I would not have to look at the revolting mess.

Sister descended on me wrathfully, about ten minutes later.

'Why haven't you eaten your lunch?' she demanded belligerently.

'I really couldn't, Sister. I don't think I could manage anything at the moment, actually, but certainly not *that*.'

'I suppose it's not good enough for you.' She gave a derogatory sniff. 'Some of you pampered women should learn not to be so fussy — there are hundreds of poor people who would be only too glad of such a meal.'

Possibly she was right, although I could not help thinking they would have to be pretty hungry actually to *enjoy* it. And what was all this 'pampered' stuff? As a family, we weren't exactly well-off ourselves and only just managed to get by on my husband's salary. I was not a fussy eater at all — but there are limits to human endurance!

'How do you expect to co-operate and do your share of the work without a good meal inside you?' She waited while I concentrated on the next contraction. 'Come along now, and be sensible; I shall stand here until I have seen you eat something.'

And so she did. My feeble protests were studiously ignored. The only way to satisfy her was to force down a few mouthfuls of the nauseating mess and hope for the best.

Now, at the end of my labours, I was becoming horribly conscious of the extreme greasiness of cold boiled mutton. My stomach, coldly churning, did its best to protest.

At last my little Malayan friend arrived to take care of me.

'I wonder if perhaps — nurse, maybe I ought to have a bowl or something.' She looked at me questioningly. I explained: 'It's just possible I might be going to throw up my lunch.'

She smiled and went away. Sister immediately appeared from nowhere. It was extraordinary how she always materialised when she was *not* wanted and never when she *was*.

'Are you still fussing?' she accused. 'You should be satisfied now that you have your baby.' She moved over to my side to straighten the blanket that covered me.

I began to explain that I had sent nurse for a bowl, simply to be on the safe side. At the same time I tried to think up a polite way of saying, 'But I *haven't* got my baby — I haven't even seen her properly yet.'

The effort was too much for me. My stomach decided to make a more emphatic protest: the boiled mutton came up much quicker than it had gone down and aimed itself competently at the front of Sister's clean bib. I honestly did not intend it to happen — in fact I was extremely sorry that it had — but there was no doubt that round one had ended up heavily in my favour.

Sister's rage and my humble apologies could have been heard for miles around.

*   *   *

Later that Sunday evening I was transferred to Ward P2 (postnatal).

My companion-in-labour — who had also given birth to a little girl — went up in the lift with me, and they put us into a four-bedded side room; the other two beds remained unoccupied.

It did not take us long to make friends, as we seemed to have quite a lot in common: we had both been left unattended, almost to the moment of birth; we had each acquired a new daughter; neither of us had been allowed more than a fleeting glimpse of the baby.

My fellow-mum (Laura, by name) had finally been given a forceps delivery and was still suffering wretchedly from the after-effects. She assured me, however, that any amount of pain and discomfort would have been worth enduring, since she and her husband had been trying for almost ten years to have a baby, and had just about given up hope when she was pronounced pregnant.

It was extremely unlikely that she would be able to have any more babies, since she was now thirty-nine years old and this birth had been a very difficult one. Naturally, she was longing to see her little girl. She hoped, too, that her husband had been allowed at least a sight of the baby when he had made a flying visit to the hospital on hearing the news.

I had not yet been able to make contact with Don, although I was sure he knew by now that we had a daughter.

Visits were not allowed on Sunday evenings. I had spent the afternoon visiting-hour in the Labour Ward, and friends who arrived at the appropriate time would have found my bed empty, presumably been told the news and, hopefully, would have passed on the message.

In Ward P2 there was a 'husbands only' rule. I was not too worried about this, as I expected to return home within the next day or so, and would then be able to entertain my family and friends in comfort. I had dutifully stayed in hospital for the actual birth (much good had it done me!); now my blood pressure had returned to normal, the danger from the toxaemia had vanished and there seemed no reason why I should not spend the required number of days in my own bed.

Laura and I both felt that it was a little hard on us that we could not see our husbands until the following day. Surely the rules could have been bent just a little? After all, we *were* in a side-room, on our own, and no one in the main wards need have been any the wiser. Not that any of the other mums would have grudged us our special treatment, I am sure — quite the reverse, probably.

Having agreed that we must just accept the situation, we were still totally unable to understand why we were not allowed to see our babies either, before settling down for the night.

Having asked several of the nurses in turn and been told each time that such a thing was impossible, we had given up the idea and relapsed into an unhappy silence, when a kindly fate decided to take a hand.

The night staff came on duty and I was delighted to find that the Staff Nurse from Ante-Natal had been posted to P2. After five weeks' stay on Ward P1, I now regarded her as an old friend, and I greeted her gladly.

'Staff! How wonderful to see you! Are you really in charge here now?'

She assured me that she was, and I explained our problem.

'Well,' she considered, 'the babies *are* all tucked up and fast asleep, and I'm not *really* supposed to, but —'

Within five minutes she was back, a baby on each arm. For the first time I held my younger daughter in my arms and examined her closely. She was a good deal smaller than my other bouncing babies, but perfectly proportioned and with delicate colouring — like a porcelain figurine, with her apple blossom complexion and a soft foam of downy, blonde hair. She was absolutely gorgeous! A surge of love for her flowed warmly over me.

I could hear Laura exclaiming over her own little girl, and when Staff switched the babies so that we could have a look at each other's, I had to admit that Laura's was one of the loveliest new-born infants I had ever seen. She had the same fair colouring and pale blonde hair and her features were beautifully chiselled. Only the cruel marks of the forceps marred her perfection: a blue-purple bruise on each delicate temple.

'But there's nothing to worry about — they'll soon fade,' Staff assured us confidently.

'Poor darling,' Laura murmured sympathetically. 'I didn't realise it was probably as bad for her as it was for me.'

Reluctantly, we had to relinquish our offspring and they were whisked off once more into the nursery. However, Staff's kindness in 'bending the rules' meant that we were able to settle down contentedly for a much-needed night's rest.

Unfortunately, although Laura slept like an angel, I found myself rigidly wide awake. Some ingenious planner had dreamed up the idea of building the hospital right next to the airport, so there was a constant coming-and-going of 'planes. Having moved up to the top floor, I was much more conscious of it than I had been in previous weeks. Still full of the excitement of the last few hours, I found it almost impossible to relax, and my mind went round and round in circles. I began to think of those at home . . .

*   *   *

Donald and I had met as fellow-workers in the Pathological Department of our local hospital: he was a laboratory technician and I a secretary, but our paths crossed quite frequently and it was not long before we were spending some time together outside working hours.

In those days I was leading an extremely busy life, very much involved in amateur drama, youth activities and various other hobbies and pursuits. I had numerous friends of both sexes and we were inclined to go around in groups of four or six, changing partners from time to time. It was all very light-hearted and enjoyable.

Don was the quiet, reliable type. He was also a home-bird and did not himself indulge in many outside activities.

However, whatever the event — whether dramatic perform-ance, five-mile hike or commercial art class, he always seemed to be there at the end of the evening, waiting patiently to escort me home.

Our relationship remained pleasantly static until I was whisked away to the north of England for six months. It was 1940 and I soon found myself in the middle of the Manchester Blitz; undisturbed sleep became a thing of the past. For nights on end the city was bombed and blasted almost out of existence. My mother and I were living with my elder sister in a service flat on the top floor of a large building and it seemed sensible to spend our nights in the communal shelter in the basement. It had been specially reinforced and was designed for the exclusive use of the house-tenants.

Despite the strong walls and ceiling, I could not help wonder-ing what would happen if the building collapsed on top of us. Who would find us under all those tons of rubble?

Most of the tenants were middle-aged or elderly and I was the only teenager there. They all made a great fuss of me and were very kind, but naturally I missed my many friends, the fun of getting up our own shows and all the other interesting activities. But, most of all, I found myself missing Donald and I spent quite a lot of my evenings in writing to him.

He, in turn, wrote almost every day, sending me the latest news of what was happening at home. Southend — like so many other places on the coast — had become quite a 'ghost' town, with a large percentage of the houses and public buildings locked up and virtually abandoned in the general evacuation that had taken place. All social activities had, of course, come to a standstill.

The Battle of Britain had been raging just before we left and it was a commonplace sight to see 'dog fights' taking place directly overhead. We had all become quite blasé about it and also virtually ignored the many bombs that fell harmlessly into the celebrated Southend mud, as enemy planes — unable to penetrate the coastal defences — jettisoned their loads before returning to Germany.

Things had quietened now — although many people considered this was just the lull before the storm. However, my mother decided that the unlikely possibility of invading German troops arriving on our doorstep was preferable to the reality of the Manchester Blitz, where buildings toppled before one's eyes and the pall of smoke never seemed to lift from the city.

So, we returned home and opened up our shuttered house once again, lighting big open fires to dispel the unlived-in atmosphere and indulging in a joyous spring-clean.

Most of my friends had been evacuated to distant places or called-up for the forces. However, I still had Donald and we virtually fell into each other's arms.

I managed to get a transfer back to the Pathological Laboratory, this time as a technician, learning the job as best I could while carrying out the actual routine.

Within six months Don and I were engaged. When we married I was hastily transferred to the Accounts Department, as a hospital rule debarred husbands and wives from working together.

The War now being virtually over, people came flooding back into the town and it was quite difficult to find apartments or flats to rent. Eventually my mother discovered a large Victorian house in the centre of the town and we shared it with her, living on separate floors and being careful not to encroach on each other's privacy.

At the end of the War, my father joined us and we all lived there happily and amicably. I left my job just before our daughter, Anthea, was born, and our first son, Christopher, arrived three years later. A traumatic time followed, when my father died of cancer after long and agonising months of suffering, and we had hardly recovered from that devastating experience when my mother fell in the snow and broke her hip. She was never to recover from this accident, and became permanently bed-bound, despite several operations.

Between her spells in hospital I nursed her at home. While she was alive and in need of care and attention, we could not think of having any more babies, which resulted in a seven-year gap between the births of our two sons.

Michael was four years old when our fourth and last baby was officially confirmed as being 'on the way'. We all decided that it would be nice if it turned out to be another girl . . .

*   *   *

Next day brought with it a daunting piece of news.

I had been delighted about 'Staff's' transfer to P2 — at least it meant there would be one familiar face among all the unknown ones. I had not bargained, however, for other shifts in duty.

It was with horror, therefore, that I recognised the new Ward Sister — yes, she had been transferred from Labour to Post Natal — the Dragon herself!

We eyed each other warily, as she made her round, but exchanged no more than a chill 'Good morning'.

Visiting time approached, the babies were brought in from the nursery and at last I was able to greet Don, give him a brief resumé of what had happened over the last two days and absorb all the news from home. The boys were well, Mum-in-law was coping with the household, and Anthea had received joyfully the news of another girl — it would even up the numbers! I had promised that the choice of name would be left to her, and after toying with the possibility of Carolyn, she had finally decided upon Catherine, with Joanne for a second name as a compliment to me.

Don examined our daughter and expressed his approval.

'This one is *my* baby,' he told me, grinning wickedly. This was not intended to cast aspersions on the parentage of the others!

Being an only child himself and envying me my brother and two sisters, he had always fancied the idea of having four children. It seemed to him to be the ideal number.

I, personally, had been inclined to call a halt at three, but it seemed a pity not to give him his 'perfect family'. I loved babies anyway, and now that we had two of each sex I was more than delighted.

Don told me that everything was ready and waiting for my return home and I should expect to be discharged at any time. I could not, of course, be expected to guess what a struggle we were going to have to effect my release.

That evening, two more mothers were moved into our room. Like me, they both had other children at home, so Laura was the only truly 'new' mother.

When the time came for the final feed of the day, her little girl was not brought in with the rest of the babies. According to Staff she had developed a 'runny eye', and they were keeping her isolated in a separate nursery.

Laura was obviously slightly upset about this, and regarded the rest of us with envy, but she cheered up eventually on being assured that there was absolutely nothing to worry about.

Next day, however, her concern grew and it spread to the rest of us when the baby again did not make an appearance. Evasive answers were all we could get out of the nursing staff, and Sister seemed to be conspicuous by her absence.

The climax came after breakfast the following morning. A nurse came in and swiftly drew the curtains around Laura's bed.

We all exchanged looks of silent consternation as Sister and one of the housemen disappeared purposefully through the curtains.

No one dared voice her thoughts; all eyes were drawn relentlessly to that shrouded corner, from which only a low rumble of voices emerged.

It was all over so suddenly: just the briefest space of time, while the news was obviously broken with no attempt to cushion the blow — then the room was filled with heartrending wailing, a sound almost sub-human, utterly intolerable to bear.

I found myself shaking uncontrollably and saw my own horror mirrored on the faces of the other women. We could only guess at what had been announced, but it was not difficult to assume that the very worst had happened.

While we were still in a state of trauma, Sister and the young doctor reappeared — the latter looking white and shaken — and left the room without even a glance at the rest of us.

One of us rang her bell and a nurse appeared in the doorway but would not come into the room or answer our anxious questions; she merely shook her head awkwardly, put a finger to her lips and went away again.

I felt torn between two decisions. Was it better to respect Laura's privacy and leave her to mourn undisturbed, or to go to her and let her know that she was not completely alone in her anguish?

I felt that I wanted to put my arms round her and reassure her — although what possible comfort I had to offer I could not imagine. I had no idea at all what her beliefs might be — or even if she had any. Nowadays, I think I would know what kind of words to say to her — at that time I was at a complete loss.

It was a relief to us all when her husband came into the room, his face set in a frozen mask of grief. He disappeared behind the curtains and soon the inhuman quality disappeared from her agonised crying, although later they both wept quietly together.

We dared not communicate with each other except by meaningful glances. The babies were brought in and we fed them with a kind of desperate haste, hoping fervently that one of them would not start to whimper. Such a sound, we felt sure, would have been altogether too much for Laura to bear.

The babies were whisked up by a scared-looking probationer and hurried back to the nursery. The hospital chaplain appeared and we directed him with silent nods towards the shrouded corner bed.

More murmuring voices, more anguished sobs — but quieter ones, this time. The hours seemed to drag interminably.

Lunch was served but none of us felt inclined to eat. All the usual routines were carried out and by tea-time Laura's curtains had been opened. She was ashen, the stark planes of her face rigid with self-control, but she seemed to have come to terms with her grief.

The glances of the other women veered away and returned to her. I knew how they felt — neither wanting to stare nor to look steadfastly the other way.

She ended our embarrassment by telling us quietly what had happened.

Apparently the baby's condition had started to deteriorate almost from birth. The paediatrician diagnosed possible brain damage arising from the forceps delivery, but it was hoped that at least physically there would soon be an improvement.

As everyone was quite optimistic, neither Laura nor her husband had been informed — which seemed to me an unforgivable omission — but the baby had suddenly developed much more alarming symptoms and emergency treatment had hardly been put into practice, when she quietly gave up the struggle.

'They told me that it was a good thing.' Laura's voice was completely devoid of expression. 'She would have been quite handicapped if she had lived.' Her eyes came to life suddenly and flashed with anger. 'But she was my baby — did they think I wouldn't have wanted to look after her?'

We did our best to comfort her in our own halting fashion. I wondered how soon it would be before they allowed her to go home. Obviously they would move her into another side-room — as far away from the babies as possible — until such time as arrangements could be made for her discharge.

But such a simple solution was not forthcoming. To our utter horror, the babies were brought in to us as usual for the six o'clock feed. No one drew Laura's curtains and she was forced to watch — and we to cope with her agonised eyes. She tried hard, but this final cruelty was all too much to bear. She soon broke down completely, racked with a frenzied sobbing.

As for the rest of us, verging on post-natal depression, we joined her in her grief, holding our unfortunate babies as if they were alien monsters, our tears flowing fast.

We were all suffering, too, from a terrible — though futile — sense of guilt. All three of us had other children at home. Laura, who had waited so long for that one baby, must have been asking bitterly and in silence: why couldn't it have been one of the others?

At last the ordeal was over. The nurses who came in to collect the babies were obviously extremely concerned for all four of us, but all their sympathy and well-meant suggestions did not soften Sister's steely heart. We had to go through the same performance twice more — until Laura's husband signed her out the following day.

She came to each of us to say goodbye. I held her closely for a few moments, trying to convey, without words, all that I felt for her.

She kissed me briefly, her eyes signalling a message that she understood and appreciated my concern, then her husband wheeled her purposefully out of the door, and I never saw her again . . .

*   *   *

I have told the story of Laura's baby, not only because it was just one more painful incident that made my hospital stay such a traumatic experience, but also to highlight the coldly impersonal — even insensitive — attitude displayed by the hospital authorities at that time.

Shortly after I arrived home there was a big outcry in the local papers about the appalling state of affairs in the maternity department of that particular hospital, and literally hundreds of mothers wrote in to describe their agonising or hair-raising experiences. I did not add my complaints to theirs, although the correspondence continued relentlessly for some weeks.

I believe that, countrywide, conditions have improved somewhat in recent years, although 'occasionally one still hears disturbing stories of women being treated, at ante-natal clinics, like child-bearing machines. They are herded together like cattle, as though lacking names and personalities, with only numbers to distinguish them one from another.

Mothers still occasionally give birth in solitary confinement, if they are unlucky enough to hit on an extra-busy time or if there is a staff shortage.

It seems to me that the whole of the Maternity Service needs to be overhauled and certain standards steadfastly maintained. For where some hospitals manage the mechanics of birth so beautifully — their efficiency and skill only matched by the loving care shown to the mothers — there are as many culprits whose uncaring, disinterested attitude causes a great deal of unnecessary pain and discomfort — and even, sometimes, considerable heartbreak.

The births of my previous three children had left me with memories that were entirely happy. Now, it seemed, nothing was going right and I could find very little cause to rejoice. Yet I did not feel that I was making an unnecessary fuss or going out of my way to look for faults in the system. Some people, I know, loathe hospitals and consequently make very bad patients. I hate to make a nuisance of myself and would not like to be mentally 'black-listed' by the resident staff.

During my five-weeks' stay in Ante-Natal, I had found no grounds for complaint. In fact, I had greatly admired the way the nurses carried out necessary — and often extremely distasteful — tasks with admirable efficiency, but also with great humanity.

Despite the boring salt-free diet, the frustration of being totally confined to bed and the sweltering heat in our Goldfish Bowl, I found hospital life bearable and my only real regret was not being able to see my younger children and, of course, missing my home.

Now, in P2, I found myself greatly disturbed by what seemed to be petty restrictions and rules so rigid that none of the nurses dared even to bend them slightly — much less break them.

It would not have mattered quite so much if the effects of this inflexible routine had not been so detrimental to both mothers and babies. But I found myself growing more and more con-

cerned as my newest daughter failed to thrive in the prevailing
conditions.

The hot summer weather had turned much cooler and the
baby seemed to feel the cold; her hands and feet were often icy to
the touch and there was a decidedly purple tinge to them. I
thought of stories I had read about 'blue' babies — at the time a
condition about which the general public knew little. Could
there be some cardiac weakness — was she suffering from what
they termed a hole-in-the-heart?

She was perfectly formed, but so tiny. It seemed to me that
her grasp on life was frail.

Sister did not approve of wrapping babies in shawls. Their
coverlets were loosely laid over the sides of the outsize cot and
not tucked in at all. My baby looked completely lost in her big
bed. Our other children had always slept peacefully and contentedly; my mother had taught me the trick of wrapping them
securely in a light shawl, tucking in the ends so that they did not
come undone. 'They feel as though they're being held in loving
arms,' she had commented and she was evidently right, because
it worked.

This baby was denied such comfort. On two occasions when
she was fretful, I lifted her out and wrapped one of the light
coverings around her, popping her back in the cot and then
laying the top cover over the high bars in the required fashion.

She slept peacefully and deeply until my dastardly act was
discovered! On the first occasion, one of the student nurses saw
what I had done and hastily undid the good work.

'Sister wouldn't approve of that at all,' she told me, scan-
dalised.

The second time, I was caught out by Sister herself.

'We don't do things in that way,' she told me, with exaggerated patience, as though trying to explain to a rather
backward five-year-old.

She, too, painstakingly put everything back the way it had
been. On both occasions the baby cried heartrendingly for a
very long time.

It was the same when it came to her feeds. The time limit —

'five minutes for each side' — was strictly adhered to. It did not matter a scrap if you had a greedy baby who gulped down all that was going in the first few minutes, or if your baby was lazy and took his time. Feeds were timed rigidly and woe betide the infant who did not conform.

Cathy, unfortunately, fell into the latter category. She did not have the strong, vigorous suck of many of the other babies. After only a minute or so, she gave up the battle and usually fell into a deep sleep. All attempts to waken her proved fruitless and, even if she could be persuaded to open her eyes, nothing would make her finish her meal.

Never had I believed more vehemently in the truth of the old adage, 'you can take a horse to water, but you can't make it drink!'

The consequence was, unfortunately, that half-an-hour after feeding-time was over I would hear her desolate wail issuing from the nursery. She had a very distinctive cry and I could always recognise it.

All pleas on my part to give her another chance were firmly refused. Sister stated, tight-lipped, that being deprived would teach her to do better next time. It seemed highly unlikely to me that a baby of only a few days would be capable of making a logical deduction from a series of facts and I was evidently right about this, for by the time the next feed came round she had cried herself into an exhausted sleep and the whole wretched cycle started over again.

Twice, at the end of the day, when the ward had settled down into a nocturnal silence — punctuated only by the distant wails of unsatisfied babies — I by-passed the night-nurse at her green-shaded desk and crept down the corridor to the nursery.

It took only a moment to whisk up my unhappy daughter and steal away to the bathroom where I could lock myself in a cubicle and feed her in peace. Strangely enough, these were the only times when she suckled contentedly and settled down happily afterwards. I suppose it might have been because of the lack of tension on my own part. A toilet seat may not have been the ideal place to nurse a baby, but at least I was not conscious of someone, stop-watch in hand, virtually breathing down my neck.

However, such pleasurable moments of togetherness were in the minority and I felt a rising sense of panic whenever I observed the fragility of Cathy's appearance, the transparent look of her skin, her tiny, blue-tinged feet.

'I don't believe we'll ever get her out of this place alive,' I told Don at the next visiting-hour. He shared my concern and set about trying to arrange my release.

On looking back, I sometimes wonder if Sister suspected that Cathy might be a mongol (the term 'Down's Syndrome' was then unknown). It would certainly account for the tenacious grasp they kept on us both, insisting that I could not be discharged without the consent of the Senior Paediatrician, who was at present on holiday. Excuse after excuse was trotted out and, baulked at every turn, I began to feel as though I were trying to escape from Colditz.

Finally my own doctor returned from leave and effected my release. On the morning of my departure, Staff Nurse appeared and explained that I might not be able to take Cathy home with me, as she had a 'sticky eye.'

I had heard this excuse before. I thought of Laura's baby and my stomach gulped coldly with fear. Even if I had to make a dash for the nursery and run down the corridor with the baby in my arms, I was determined to get her out of this place without delay.

However, such drastic steps proved unnecessary. Don arrived, with our doctor in tow, and gently but firmly insisted on my discharge.

Sister came to me as I was leaving and, to my utter astonishment, apologised quietly for having caused me any distress during my labour and subsequent stay on her ward. On reflection, I am now almost certain that she foresaw my child's handicap and envisaged all the difficulties it would create. It was pity that forced an apology from her and not a complete change of heart.

I have never asked for pity and would not have wanted it

then, even if I had known what was in her mind; but I wish that she had told me of her suspicions. Even a hint on her part would have saved me so much soul-searching later on.

Chapter 2

It was wonderful to be home again. After an ecstatic reunion I sat like some old mother hen, with the children gathered round me, wishing that I had more than the allotted one pair of arms.

Michael was the only one to hold back at first, shrinking away against his grandmother's comforting frame and staring at me in silence.

I had taken particular care not to have the baby in my arms when I first greeted him, not wanting him to think of her as a usurper, ousting him from his rightful place. She had been placed straight into her cot upon arrival.

I was puzzled and not a little hurt, having expected him to rush forward and half-strangle me with the intensity of his welcome. Curbing the strong desire to sweep him up into my arms and hold him tightly, I simply smiled brightly and continued to ask him polite questions about his doings at school.

The wall of separation lasted for about ten minutes, then he ran forward and flung himself on to my lap, bursting into floods of tears. After a warm cuddle and lots of reassurance, we were 'friends' again.

It was not for some years that I learned exactly how much he had suffered during my prolonged absence.

When we had known for sure that I was being shipped into hospital, Donald and I had given much thought to the best way of breaking the news to Michael. The others were old enough to understand what was happening and to accept the fact that hospitalisation was a necessary evil, but at four years old, the current 'baby' of the family, he could not be expected to react in the same way.

We decided finally that it would not be a good idea to tell him before he left home in the morning. He was beginning to settle down well at school, enjoying his day's activities, and it might surely do a great deal of harm to let him spend a whole day worrying about what was happening to me. We both felt it would be much better for Don to explain about it on the way home and to prepare him gently for the fact that I would not be in the house to greet him.

It turned out to be a very bad decision on our part. Although he gave no outward sign of his feelings, Michael was quite convinced in his own mind that I had died during the day and had been hastily smuggled out of the house and buried, all the talk of my staying in hospital being a fabrication for the sole purpose of keeping the news of my death from him!

Although quite amusing to look back on, this conviction must have been totally shattering for him. It is only incredible that no one realised what was going on in his child's mind.

'But what about the times I spoke to you on the 'phone?' I asked.

'I thought they had got someone to pretend to be you.'

'And the cards and letters I sent you?'

'I was sure those had been sent by someone else, too.' He grinned. 'Don't forget, Mum, I was only four and I couldn't recognise your handwriting.'

I was thunderstruck.

'But how dreadfully cruel you must have felt everyone was being, to do such a thing.'

'Not a bit. I thought they were all trying to be very kind.'

It just shows that, however good the relationship, we do not really know what is going on in our children's minds . . .

But now we were all together again, and things would be just as they were before — with the addition of a new member of the family, of course.

'Mum, I fell out of a tree and busted my finger,' reported our accident-prone elder son, not without a certain relish. 'I had to go to the hospital but they said it wasn't broken. Or even discollated,' he added, almost regretfully.

'Discollated — you mean dislocated.' This from his sister, somewhat scathingly. 'Don't you know the Queen's English?'

'Of *course* I do — else she wouldn't be Queen of England, would she?'

Hoots of laughter all round.

Our younger son slid off my lap and went over to the cot, peering in curiously.

'She's a very *little* baby,' he decided finally. 'Will she be able to play with me?'

'Not for a while,' I told him. 'She doesn't know how to do very much yet.'

'I'll teach her,' he said stoutly.

We did not know at the time how prophetic those words were to be.

*   *   *

It did not take long for us to slip back into the old routine and it seemed almost as though I had never been away. My mother-in-law, who had come to look after the household for what we hoped would be only a few days and had manfully stuck it out for almost six weeks, now returned home and I took up the reins once again.

Right from the start, Cathy fitted into our family pattern beautifully. Now that we were freed from the rigid hospital routine, I had no problems with her feeding and, with that difficulty out of the way, everything else seemed to fall into place quite naturally.

She was such a good baby: sleeping sixteen hours out of the twenty-four, waking, taking her feed like an angel, then rewarding me with a brief, sweet smile before relapsing into sleep again.

In the light of present-day knowledge, of course, we were doing all the wrong things. Current practice with mentally handicapped children is to keep them stimulated continuously from birth, not allowing them to fall into bad habits where their mental processes are concerned.

Fortunately, her placid routine caused no permanent damage, as far as it is possible to tell — although with the prescribed treatment she might have made a much earlier start.

As it was, I was extremely thankful that she was such a model baby. I went back to my job on Listener Research for the BBC. It involved calling on people in their homes and asking them about the TV programmes they had seen. The baby went with me in her Karri-Cot and slept happily through most of the interviews.

We would finish the afternoon by collecting Michael from school, getting home in good time for Family Tea (one always seemed to think of it in capital letters!), when we all congregated together and spent a happy — and often hilarious — hour reviewing the events of everyone's day.

After that, Anthea took over. She had virtually adopted the baby and took a delight in bathing, dressing and feeding her, before putting her into that invaluable Karri-Cot on wheels and going out for a short walk — by which time Cathy was fast asleep and ready to be tucked down for the night.

It provided a useful interval in which I was able to supervise Michael's bath, spare him half-an-hour's 'mothering' time and finish up by reading a story to him in bed. By the time we reached the end he was virtually falling asleep — although protesting drowsily that he was not!

This routine followed a pattern we had always adhered to. With the advent of each new baby, we felt it was important not to neglect the next-in-age, the child who had previously *been* the cosseted baby. He or she should be shown that Mum still wanted to share in their 'special hour' and would fiddle the time-table somehow to provide for it. In this way we had always been able to avoid the dangers of jealousy and resentment. I am a firm believer in the principle (now considered 'old fashion'), that if parents spent just a little more time with their children, showed just a little more genuine interest, half the present-day juvenile problems would be solved.

With Anthea and Cathy off for the evening walk and Michael and myself totally absorbed in the awful doings of Mr Toad or Peter Rabbit, Christopher and Don knuckled down to the serious business of model-making or taking clocks to pieces to see how they worked. There was just time to fit in such a session before Don had to leave for the theatre. He had resigned from his job as a laboratory technician some time before, when our voluntary hospital had been taken over by the State and everything tied up in a smothering mass of red tape — even the simplest of requests having to be made in triplicate. He was now resident Stage Manager at the local repertory theatre, his years of work with amateur drama groups finally paying dividends.

We might well have continued following this idyllic family routine in blissful ignorance, but somewhere in the back of my mind there niggled the strong conviction that something was wrong with the baby.

Everyone was very patient with me and suggested gently that perhaps I was still suffering from the after-effects of my stay in hospital. After all, I had had five weeks before the birth, when my health had caused some concern and the toxaemia had waged a relentless battle with my protesting system. Following this, there was the trauma of the actual birth and my anxiety for the baby's welfare afterwards. It wasn't surprising, was it, that I should feel a little depressed and under the weather?

Somehow I could not make anyone understand that I was not simply suffering from depression, and as for being 'under the weather' — well, physically I had really no complaints. It was just that somehow, deep within me, I *knew* that all was not well — the only thing I could not fathom was what the actual problem might be. Cathy, meanwhile, continued to thrive, to put on weight and to show every sign of become a model child.

There were two very disturbing occasions, however, when all was very definitely *not* well with her.

As it happened, on both occasions Anthea and I were alone with the baby, Don having taken the boys out for the afternoon.

That first time, I was totally unprepared for what was to come. The baby, who had been lying happily in her pram, suddenly gave a kind of choking gurgle and when I turned to find out if she had perhaps vomited some of her feed, I was disturbed to see every vestige of colour slowly draining from her face. It was more than just a question of 'turning pale'. I have witnessed the ghastly pallor of patients suffering from a massive blood-loss and the deathly whiteness of someone in deep shock, but nothing like that could compare with the absolute bloodlessness of my baby's face — even her lips were totally and undeniably white.

I snatched her up out of the pram, calling to Anthea to fill a hot-water bottle quickly. I cannot describe the horrific sensation I experienced when I took the small body into my arms. It was just as though every bone had turned to jelly — she was completely limp and flaccid — but again it was like nothing I had experienced before, nor have done since.

As though in a nightmare, I went through all the correct actions, but when there was no response, as a last resort I put the baby down on to the table and proceeded to carry out the resuscitation treatment commonly known as the 'kiss of life'.

Within minutes I felt a faint movement, saw the rib-cage rise and fall and was suddenly aware of the firm bones in her body again. She gave a gasp, then an enormous kind of belch and the colour came flooding back into her face.

It was quite extraordinary, but five minutes later she looked and felt completely normal. She even laughed up at me, as though she had been teasing us all the time. By now, Anthea had put through an emergency call to our doctor. Since the latter lived only in the next road she came round immediately. Of course, I was full of apologies, since Cathy now looked none the worse for her experience — in fact I think *we* were the ones who felt we needed treatment!

Fortunately our doctor knew me well and realised that I would certainly not have sent for her light-heartedly. Nevertheless, she found it as difficult to understand the symptoms as I found it to describe them. She carried out a thorough examination then and there, but could find no possible cause for such a happening. It had certainly been no ordinary convulsion, I knew, nor even some kind of fit, for I had had plenty of experience of both.

By this time, Don and the boys had returned home and I felt

almost sheepish as I tried to explain exactly why I had called out the doctor on a Sunday afternoon!

When the same thing happened again, just a few weeks later, I was not taken so completely by surprise but, of course, at the first sign of distress — that terrible 'draining' of the blood from face and lips — I was engulfed by a great rush of fear, dreading what I knew was to come.

Once again, total collapse seemed to follow and that horrific sensation of holding a body from which all the bones had been removed. Her shallow breathing seemed to stop almost immediately, but this time I was ready for it and embarked immediately on resuscitation action. While Anthea ran for hot water, I began to give the kiss of life. Recovery took place as before, the colour slowly washing back into her waxen lips and cheeks.

There were no more infantile attacks after this, although during her early years Cathy appeared to 'faint' several times, with very similar effects. Despite various tests and an extremely thorough examination by a distinguished and most interested consultant, no one has ever found a satis-factory explanation.

As she has matured, the intervals between these strange attacks have lengthened: first a year's gap, then two years and now I am thankful to say she has had no return of the symptoms for five or six years.

However, I found the two earliest experiences extremely disquieting and it has since occurred to me that, had she been in bed at the time — alone at night — there would probably have been one more unexplained 'cot death' in our locality. As it was, I offered up a grateful prayer of thanks that I had been close at hand and had sufficient knowledge to bring her virtually back to life.

I feel very strongly that every responsible person should learn how to carry out the kiss of life procedure. It is such a simple technique to master, but in an emergency it might well spell the difference between life and death.

Shortly after this, I found myself endorsing my opinion at our

annual Town Show. This ambitious venture was staged over
three or four days in one of the largest of our local parks, where
a number of outsize marquees housed booths and stalls representing various aspects of Southend life.

For example, there were agricultural displays by all the
horticultural societies and floral arrangement clubs in the town;
fur and feather competitions; dog and cat shows; a military
tattoo organised by the local barracks; musical and dramatic
performances; a trading exhibition; handicraft entries and
many, many other things.

We were helping in the Social Services marquee. This had
nothing to do with the Government department of that name,
but consisted of booths and displays related to various charities,
local churches, youth groups and such facilities as the Lifeboat
Service, Red Cross and Animal Welfare Services.

We found it an interesting experience and stayed on duty for
most of the time, packing enough food for the day and anything
else we were likely to need.

Cathy was as happy and contented as usual in her Karri-Cot
and stayed with us on our pitch, except for an occasional airing
outside. Anthea, too, preferred to help man the booth. The boys
had a whale of a time visiting all the other marquees and
making themselves useful on the field.

It was while I was making a tour of the other exhibits in our
tent, Cathy in my arms, that I encountered a member of the St
John Ambulance Brigade giving a demonstration of how to
perform the kiss of life.

He had drawn quite a little crowd of people about him and
was urging them to learn the correct method so that they might
be ready to help in a possible emergency.

There were some rather scathing and facetious comments
being bandied to and fro and he was not really having much of a
success.

I was extremely sorry for the poor man and, despite misgivings, I felt compelled to move through the crowd and stand
at his side.

'He's absolutely right,' I heard myself announcing firmly. 'If

I hadn't known exactly what to do, this baby wouldn't be alive today.'

The crowd turned and viewed us with interest.

'It's true,' I went on hastily, although I was really quite taken aback at my own intervention, 'I don't belong to the Ambulance Brigade and I'm no kind of expert, but I just happened to have been taught by a friend how to do the right thing.'

I recounted what had happened and the crowd seemed to be quite impressed. Afterwards, the St John's man thanked me.

'Do you think you could do that again next time I demonstrate?' he asked enthusiastically. 'We could work up quite a performance between us!'

I wasn't at all sure that was such a good idea. What had been a spontaneous urge on my part probably wouldn't come over quite so well if it were pre-arranged and carefully rehearsed.

However, I was quite happy to agree to his referring to our particular experience and for the rest of the day I could hear his 'spiel' floating across the marquee:

'. . . And that young lady over there can vouch for what I am saying. Why, that sweet little baby wouldn't be here today if somebody hadn't happened to show . . .'

There was a booth quite near to ours which filled me with an intense feeling of depression every time I passed it. Posters of sad-eyed children, their faces half-shadowed, provided a sombre background for the display-table which was stacked with pathetic bundles of wood, presumably packed by similar children. I knew it was the stand allotted to the local Society for the Mentally Handicapped.

It aroused no other emotion within me, except deep sympathy. I did not feel the need to approach those on duty or ply them with questions; I simply bought a few bundles of wood and dropped the change I was given into the accompanying collecting-box. It was merely a gesture of compassion, made almost with embarrassment, for what else was there for me to do? Such children did not enter into our own happy little world.

Perhaps I should have enquired more closely; but the

stirrings of disquiet that I felt about our own baby were all allied to physical causes. Not for a moment had I ever considered that we might be the parents of a mentally handicapped child.

*   *   *

Enlightenment came to me in a totally shattering way.

Months had passed and my earlier fears for Cathy had dimmed somewhat. Although her progress was slow compared to that of my other children at the same age, I had come to accept the advice of a friendly neighbour who had remonstrated with me: 'The other three were all so very forward for their ages. It's not fair to compare her to them; children mature at different rates. This one probably prefers to take her time.'

I still wondered sometimes if there might not be some slight physical weakness, and I used to massage her limbs daily and play little games to help her to exercise them. She seemed thoroughly to enjoy my ministrations but was not much inclined to make any efforts of her own. However, I decided that I must not try to hurry her. I should let her take as much time as she wanted.

Her first birthday came and passed. One day, I was browsing round our local Woolworth's store, with Cathy in her push-chair, when I met an old friend whom I had not seen for years.

After exchanging greetings and swapping news of our respective families, she glanced down at Cathy.

'And this is your latest, is it?' Her expression altered slightly, then she said in a bright but casual manner: 'Oh, she's a little mongol, bless her!'

I stared at her, shock, like an icy hand, clutching at my heart.

'No — no — she's not!' I heard myself stammering.

'Oh, but she is, love. I've been working with them for years and there's no mistaking —' She evidently read and understood the expression on my face. 'Oh, Lord! Hadn't they told you? I'm so sorry —'

I mumbled something unintelligible, turned and stumbled blindly out of the store into the harsh, unsympathetic brightness of the sunlight outside. It took me only five minutes to reach home, running all the way.

Once indoors, I automatically put on the kettle ready for tea. Then I snatched up the baby and held her closely to me, wrapping my arms tightly around her as though by this very action I could shield her from the world.

Although one part of me had not yet fully accepted the nature of her true disability, my other self was already anticipating with sick dread the difficulties she and the rest of the family would surely have to face.

Slowly, the cold, numb feeling melted. To be able to cry would have been such a relief, but I was caught up in an anguish too deep for tears.

The whistle of the kettle brought me back to the realities of daily living. Soon the children would be in for tea and I had to be able to put on my normal, welcoming face; to meet them with cheerfulness; to listen to their eager outpourings of the day's happenings.

What I must *not* do was share my sense of grief and shock with them. Above everything else I longed to communicate with someone — anyone — to offload the intolerable burden on to someone else's shoulders. But, however strong the temptation, I knew that I could not, without warning, inflict such pain on the members of my own family. At any rate, not yet.

I would have to choose the right time and use the right words and attempt to soften the blow as much as I possibly could.

But the right time never seemed to materialise. Days — and then weeks — went by and I was still carrying the burden alone. I had tried to explain the position to Don, but he shied away from my fumbled words. He assured me that I was jumping to wild conclusions. What did a member of the general public really know about such things? Maybe she *had* put in a little work with mongol children, but it didn't make her an expert — and if her diagnosis were a true one, why hadn't one of the doctors said anything to us?

It was the first time that I had ever turned to my husband for support, only to meet with what seemed to be an invisible brick wall between us. He did not want to consider the possibility of Cathy being handicapped and therefore studiously avoided all discussion of the subject. I could not understand his attitude at all, but I was later to find out that this was a typical reaction on the part of the father.

Although it was not so in every case, a good many mothers — once they had emerged from their first shocked state — accepted the diagnosis, listened to whatever advice was available and then, for better or worse, set out to bring up their handicapped child in the best way they could manage — making allowances, of course, for the degree of retardation.

A large percentage of the fathers, however, found the situation almost impossible to accept — in fact, in many cases, they utterly refused to admit to the child's subnormality.

I was later to find that many of the men who served with me on mental handicap committees and were without doubt our most tireless and devoted workers, had initially refused even to join the local Society, since this would have meant admitting that their child had a handicap.

It was certainly unusual in those days to find fathers of *young* children turning up to help at functions where the handicapped might be found *en masse*. Only after a period of time, when he had managed to accept the inevitable and learned to live with it, did the average father suddenly emerge from the shadows and take his place among the other workers.

Nowadays, of course, when so much early counselling takes place and sympathetic support is offered to new parents, the 'dads' are as much in evidence at meetings as the 'mums' — perhaps even more so.

But for me, at that time, it was a daunting experience, and for quite a while it prevented me from approaching any other member of my family. Had my parents still been living, I think it would have been a very different story. My sisters had moved away from the immediate vicinity and it was not a subject I felt could be tackled by letter or on the 'phone.

The only other person I might have confided in was Anthea, and I shrank from causing her any kind of distress. She was only in her 'teens and her delight and interest in this long-awaited little sister were so rewarding to watch. I thought of the bond between myself and my eldest sister (there was just about the same age-gap) and remembered our perfect relationship when I had been a child. Somehow I could not break into their happy little world — not until I was really sure.

But in my heart I knew that I had found out the truth. Hugging the knowledge to myself, in the loneliness of my anguish, it was difficult to know where to go for help.

I visited the local library and searched the shelves until I found a book dealing with the subject of mongolism. It was not at all helpful as far as offering advice was concerned. It laid down no rules for me to follow, gave no indication of how I could help to stimulate that slumbering mind. It did, however, show me how to recognise a mongol baby (for example, the 'fold' at the inner corner of the eye) and I knew then, without doubt, that my friend had diagnosed Cathy's condition correctly.

The ponderous chapters held out no hope for the future. My child, I was told, was 'ineducable'; she would be incapable of being toilet-trained; I could count myself lucky if she were able to learn a few simple words — but if she talked at all, her speech would be slurred and delivered in a gruff and guttural tone. The only comfort offered seemed to be that mongol children were usually placid in disposition, affectionate and amenable to commands — providing, of course, they understood them.

A footnote added that they seldom lived beyond their 'teens, being highly susceptible to chest and other infections. The author seemed to look upon this final piece of information as a kind of bonus — a sugar coating to sweeten the pill. (With any luck, you won't have to put up with it for long, dear.)

I was incensed and more than shocked, and I think the information went a long way towards helping me to make up my mind. I knew I was in for a fight and the more I thought about it the stronger my determination grew.

I examined my baby with her soft, fair curls, her skin with the delicate fragile look of English porcelain and the sweet, fleeting smile with which she rewarded me when I spoke to her. Could I imagine her growing up into the kind of child described in that most frightening book — short and squat, with a shuffling gait, stubby fingers and a tongue that lolled permanently out of a loose, drooling mouth?

It seemed impossible that such a transformation could take place. Had not my sister, when visiting, said that this was the prettiest of all my babies?

Yet undoubtedly I had seen such children as those featured in the book; they were usually being towed along in the wake of elderly parents and casual passers-by averted their eyes, feeling uncomfortable in their presence. Now, perhaps, in my turn I would have to face the embarrassment or, worse, the open stares of other people.

One thing was certain. I had to emerge from my private world of grief and shock and take up the challenge; steel myself to let our daughter be seen without shame or apology.

I would not try to hide her if she were blind or deaf or had difficulty in walking — why, then, should she be hidden because she was mentally, instead of physically, handicapped?

All the same, I was going to need help. Somewhere there must be a better source of information than that infamous book. After all, there were other mothers with children like mine . . .

Suddenly I recalled our neighbouring booth at the Town Show. I could visualise again the posters with the sad-eyed children, the piled-up bundles of wood. Somewhere in the town there was an Association that dealt with such things.

I grabbed up the 'phone-book and anxiously riffled through the pages. Yes, there it was: Southend and District Society for Mentally Handicapped Children.

With fingers that had grown suddenly unaccountably clumsy, I lifted the 'phone and dialled the number. There was no answer and immediately a rush of relief flooded over me. It is difficult to explain this reaction, but although I needed help and was anxious to talk to *someone*, at the same time I dreaded putting my fears into words. And how was I to begin? What exactly did I want to say to this faceless stranger?

I tried twice more, at intervals, but without success. In the unreasonable way that we humans behave, I now felt aggrieved that I had been unable to make contact.

Noting the address listed in the 'phone-book, I wrote to the Society asking for details of how to join. A few days later, a note was pushed through my door. (How I would have welcomed a *call* from a fellow-parent and a few reassuring words.) A meeting was to be held the following week, when a visiting speaker would be talking about some of the problems families of handicapped children have to face.

*   *   *

I went alone, and sat at the back of the drab, depressing hall. No one came up to speak to me or acknowledge my presence. Up on the platform, someone read out a few notices about unpaid subscriptions and the need for more jumble for a forthcoming sale, then introduced the speaker, a bright-faced woman with a chirpy voice that was so unbelievably artificial it gave me the nightmare feeling that I was watching Joyce Grenfell in cabaret.

During the next half-hour she trotted out all the classic problems I had read about in my book and added a good many more to the list. Her delivery was arch and her manner half-apologetic, half-bracing, as though she were a disappointed teacher encouraging a class of apathetic children to do better.

No attempt was made to suggest any ways of combating such problems; the sole purpose of the talk was apparently to armour us parents against the very difficult times to come. The general message seemed to be: 'don't fight it, just accept it and submit'.

Questions were then invited and our speaker let her gaze rove hopefully over the audience, flashing an over-bright smile in our general direction.

There were no questions. I think everyone was too despondent to want to discuss the matter, and they had my sympathy. I think I might have had a question or two of my own if I had not been quite certain that no helpful answers would be forthcoming.

The whole thing finally petered out and we were told that tea and biscuits would now be served. I would have left there and then but felt it was hardly fair to condemn the entire Society on the strength of one wasted evening. I looked around me, hoping to find some kindred soul — some new parent like myself, feeling her way. There were one or two small groups of people standing about, but each seemed to be eyeing the others almost with suspicion; there was no appearance of togetherness or comradeship.

Feeling like a fish out of water, I asked a woman who was walking round with a tray of tea: 'Could you tell me how I can find out more about the Society, please?'

She stared at me as though I had suggested something obscene.

'Well — I really couldn't say. Our Chairman isn't here this evening; that's the Secretary over there — perhaps she can help you.'

The Secretary, who seemed to be surrounded by miscellaneous papers and looked totally distraught, gazed at me speechlessly for a moment and then asked distractedly: 'What exactly was it you wanted to know? We are having another speaker soon and I believe there's an outing being planned . . . Perhaps you'd better leave your name and address.'

I did not bother to tell her that she already had it. How else would I have known about tonight's meeting?

'Can I join the Society?' At least that would be a start.

This seemed to upset her even more.

'Oh, dear — I don't know. Our Treasurer's here somewhere, but I can't see him at the moment. Perhaps you'd better sit down and wait . . .' She turned away as someone buttonholed her on the other side.

This was it, then. No welcome; no enquiries about my child or questions as to what form her handicap might take. No help.

I walked away and left the building without speaking to anyone else.

On the way home I tried to sort out my tempestuous thoughts. Perhaps I *had* been mistaken after all to try to fight the inevitable. Perhaps tonight's speaker had been right and I should simply submit uncomplainingly to what was to come. What right had I to think that I knew better than all the experts?

Having reached home, I just could not bring myself to go into the house. Don was still at the theatre, the children were all in bed. I knew the friend who was acting as baby-sitter would not be expecting to see me for a while. Somehow I could not face her cheery greeting and the half-an-hour or so of bright conversation over the inevitable cup of tea.

I walked up and down the street outside the house, crying inwardly and praying silently for someone, somewhere to help me. But although my prayers were sincere as well as desperate I was not, at that time, truly aware of the closeness of God. I had never felt so alone in my whole life.

Reaching the gate once more, I put my hand on the latch, knowing that it was no use postponing the evil hour any longer; I could not stay out in the dark on my own for ever.

Suddenly, I was acutely aware of my mother's presence. There was no ghostly manifestation, but in my mind's eye I could see her face clearly and she was looking at me with an expression in which I could read sadness and love and a deep compassion.

I had seen that look once before and the memory of it was like a revelation to me. The surge of feeling that washed over me at that moment was so overwhelming that I felt physically faint. I clung to the gate as though it were a lifeline, until the unpleasant symptoms receded and my legs felt less as though they were made of indiarubber.

I had my answer. Why on earth had I not seen the parallel before? I knew now that I would go on and fight and, God willing, win. Because, of course, history was about to repeat itself . . .

*   *   *

I was the fourth child born to my parents and something of an 'after-thought', since they were both over forty and my brother and sisters respectively seven, ten and fourteen years older than myself.

Surrounded by love, I was very much the pampered baby of the family, but I do not think I ever became 'spoilt' — my elder brother saw to that! He was my idol and my constant companion once I was old enough to go out and about with him.

I have often thought since that it must have been a bit of a trial for his friends always to have a small sister trailing along behind, but they certainly seemed to accept me affably enough and I was included in all their games and adventures. It was a very good training-ground as, naturally, I was expected to behave in the same way as all the boys. Cut knees, bruised heads and other damages were taken in my stride; no tears were allowed and whining strictly forbidden.

In between these tough male pursuits, I learned from my sisters to play with dolls and all the other occupations favoured by small girls. They also loved to dress me up in pretty clothes and take me to interesting places.

More than anything, though, I remember our oneness as a family. Despite the difference in ages we were at our happiest when we were all together and there always seemed to be such intriguing things to do.

My father was a gentle, kindly man. I cannot remember hearing him raise his voice in anger to anyone, yet we would not have dreamt of disobeying him, nor did other people take advantage of him; he was always greatly admired and respected.

My mother was a more volatile character but she had great charm and warmth and what was then called 'personality'. Even when she was elderly, people loved to spend time in her company and young people particularly adored her. When, after we were married, Donald and I had gatherings of friends in our part of the house, it was a foregone conclusion that some of them would disappear for part of the evening. We knew we could always find them in Mother's flat, revelling in her company.

Both my parents were artistically inclined; my father had a delightful singing voice and also played the zither and my mother was a very talented pianist. They were much in demand in the days when musical evenings were in vogue and, of course, music was an important part of my childhood background. Added to this, my father wrote poetry and composed songs — although purely for his own amusement.

From quite an early age I made up my mind that I wanted to go on the stage when I was old enough. We were always getting up shows and putting on plays; we had a large trunkful of dressing-up clothes and quite a bit of talent between us. My sister Elsie had a lovely voice, Mary was the dancer of the family and we could all act. We usually wrote our own shows and enticed in anyone we could get hold of to watch the production. Having no audience, however, was no deterrent and at such times we simply performed for our own pleasure.

When we were not striding the boards ourselves we would put on plays or concerts in our toy theatre, with cardboard characters that were pushed on from the sides of the stage on long wires. My brother John had been given a most ingenious torch that could be switched on to shine red, white or green and it made a marvellous coloured spotlight.

Sometimes we would rig up a sheet with a lamp behind it and give a shadow-show. We were always trying out new devices, but when the four of us were together the majority of our games were geared towards 'showbiz'.

Our parents had always been extremely keen on the theatre and had introduced that magic world to us at an early age — an example I followed later with our own children.

By the time I was entering my 'teens, it was an accepted fact that when I was old enough I would go to drama school. I was already attending dancing and drama classes and often filled the breach in local entertainment circles when a solo act was needed. All this, added to our own home-made productions, kept me very happy until something happened that changed my whole way of life.

I had just settled in at a new school when I developed what

was at first supposed to be a 'weak ankle'. While I was taking part in games or gym, it constantly crumpled under me and let me down; I also found that there were certain basic dancing-steps I could no longer perform properly. I began to find this disability very tiresome and even a little disturbing; but I managed to hide it from my mother, as I felt sure she would whip me off somewhere for advice and I simply hated going to doctors.

Eventually our gym-mistress noticed that I seemed to be dragging my right foot; she sent for my mother and an emergency appointment was made with a local specialist, who confirmed my teacher's suspicions by announcing that I had contracted polio myelitis or — as it was more generally called in those days — infantile paralysis.

This disease was then almost unheard-of and there had been very few cases recorded in Essex, although very soon after this it became a considerable scourge and crippled and even killed hundreds of children and adults alike. But at the time I contracted it, nothing much had been discovered in the way of treatment. There were, of course, no vaccines and the only known way of dealing with polio was complete bedrest with absolute immobilisation of the affected limb. If you were lucky, this usually isolated the trouble in one particular part of your body, leaving your other limbs unaffected; if you were not, then the deadly disease spread rapidly and if it reached your diaphragm or lungs you would probably die of asphyxiation as the paralysis prevented normal respiration.

I was terrified of being sent to what was then referred to as the Fever Hospital — a very ancient building about which I had heard some hair-raising stories. Knowing this, my mother dug in her heels and put up a terrific fight until the authorities reluctantly agreed to let her nurse me at home.

'You do realise you are running a great risk of catching it yourself?' they warned her.

My mother scorned the idea. She had nursed my sisters through diphtheria and scarlet-fever — after having had the same stand-up fight with authority — and staunchly believed that if you were not afraid of a disease you could not catch it. Seeing that she had had experience in fever-nursing and knew all the correct procedures, they finally agreed to her wishes and I was hastily shipped home and isolated in a room at the top of the house, with 'fever-sheets' hung around the door.

I was put to bed, surrounded by unwieldy sandbags which were supposed to keep me immobilised. They certainly helped to do this but they were intolerably hot and scratchy, even after my mother made linen cases to slip over them.

A time of nightmare followed. Weeks of lying on my back and not being able to do any of the things I most enjoyed — except reading, of course. Fortunately I had always been a bookworm and this occupation kept me sane. My mother spent as much time with me as she could, but she had a large house to run and a family to look after and cook, wash and shop for.

One day she had an ingenious idea and rigged up a mirror that would catch the reflections of people passing in the street below, so that at least I had something other than four walls to watch. Shades of the Lady of Shallot!

It seemed a very long and tedious time, with no visitors allowed and all movements curtailed. I missed my brother and sisters very much but felt a great deal happier when they decided to publish a weekly magazine for me, with contributions from all the family. This consisted of puzzles, stories, jokes and a very exciting serial entitled 'The Mysterious Schoolgirl'. It was written in penny exercise books and copiously illustrated, and each week I looked forward eagerly to publication day. I still have those magazines and occasionally re-read them and find them very entertaining!

At last the period of isolation was over. Although I was still not allowed to move my legs, at least I could be propped up into a sitting position. This gave me much more scope and I could now do such things as jigsaw puzzles — although I must have been a sore trial to my long-suffering mother as I was always dropping vital pieces, and of course I was not allowed to lean out of bed to pick them up. All I could do was ring the bell to summon her aid.

She must have looked forward to the day when I would be on my feet again; but that was still far in the future. At the end of the 'quiescent' period, as it was called, I was given a thorough examination, and although my doctor smiled cheerfully and assured me that everything was going well, he had to break the news to my mother that the muscle on one side of my leg was totally useless and it was extremely unlikely that I would ever walk again.

The hateful sandbags had been taken away and I was now free to move about — if I could. But my foot hung down uselessly and I could not lift it or raise my toes at all. With all the optimism of youth, I did not let this depress me too much, feeling sure that it was only a matter of time before everything would return to normal.

Appalled at the news as they were, my family managed to keep me in ignorance and put on a brave face for my benefit. One slender thread of hope was held out: that it would be possible for me to have intensive therapy to see if the useless muscle might be revitalised and made to work once again. If this treatment failed, it would mean that I would have to wear an iron calliper for the rest of my life.

There was general agreement that nothing should be reported to me until all possible treatments had been tried and found to fail. Everyone hoped desperately that such a time would never come.

It was a friend of the family who — not agreeing with their decision — felt it was his duty to tell me the truth. Baldly, without any kind of preparation and with great cruelty, he told me: 'There is no point in deceiving yourself. You will never walk again.'

I was only a child and had utterly no inkling until then of how serious my illness had been. This announcement came as a tremendous shock and sent my temperature soaring. Our doctor was puzzled by my sudden regression, for I could not bring myself to talk about it. Greatly concerned, my mother finally guessed what had happened. She immediately launched a campaign to build up my hopes again. It must have been a time of great trial for her, doing her best to encourage and cheer me, while having to face the true facts and also to offer what comfort she could to the rest of the family.

The time finally came when I could be carried downstairs in triumph. How strange the rest of the house looked after my prolonged absence, but how good it was to leave the prison of that upstairs room.

Now began a new and very wearisome routine. Three times a week my mother wheeled me in my invalid chair to the local hospital — there was no convenient transport service to take us in those days. The treatment I had to undergo was long, painful and quite soul-destroying. Massage, manipulation and electric shock treatment were interspersed with periods of being encased in a plaster cast. For eighteen months my life seemed to revolve round these sessions of physical and mental torment. I certainly learned to endure pain — and without a murmur or a tear, since that was the way I had been taught to behave — but I was too young at the time to realise what an awful ordeal it must have been for my mother. She would sit beside me during all the worst moments at the hospital, letting me grip her hand as tightly as I wanted to, and always with a smile of encouragement and just the right words to bolster me up.

Years later, she told me exactly how much she had suffered, watching her youngest child being subjected to such things and not being able to show her true feelings. She rarely slept at night and, of course, her days were long and gruelling as she strove to divide her time fairly between our hospital trips and the needs of the rest of the family.

She had always been slight in build and certainly, during the next few years, she lost even more weight, but she managed to keep going without buckling under, although she admitted much later that she rarely had time to eat a proper meal and existed mostly on toast and innumerable cups of tea.

The whole family rallied round and gave as much support as possible, though they all had exacting jobs to hold down. John and Elsie spent hours keeping me amused and took me out in my wheelchair whenever possible. My eldest sister, Mary, continually thought up new ways of taking my mind off the ordeals to come; she also supervised my neglected education and set me various lessons and exercises to perform, marking and correcting them when she came home from work in the evening and even instigating a Prize-Giving Day when I was presented with books as awards for my best efforts.

My father's job took him away for most of the time and he was able to come home only on alternate weekends. At those times he shared the burden of trying to keep me from dwelling too much on what I might next have to undergo, and would sit by me for hours singing every song in his repertoire. We also composed poems together and made up stories.

But the abortive efforts to awaken some life in my unresponding limb could not go on for ever. My mother insisted on having a second opinion and I was allowed to see a new consultant — an orthopaedic surgeon this time, who was beginning to make quite a name for himself. Mr Whitchurch-Howell: his ideas were obviously years ahead of his time.

It was long before the days of transplant surgery or joint replacement, yet he had already had great success in making a new elbow-joint for a man who had smashed his own in falling off a ladder. He had also replaced other small bones and cartilages.

He spent a good hour examining me and asking me pertinent questions. I was then left alone for a time while he was closeted with my mother.

To her he offered a difficult and frightening choice. He told her quite honestly that there was no possible chance of my regaining the use of my leg; that the muscle had atrophied beyond hope of revival and that the ordeal of the last eighteen months had been an utter waste of time.

Having dealt this body-blow he then explained the possible alternatives that would govern my future. I could be fitted with a calliper and in time I would probably be able to get about in it unaided — although always with difficulty; I could continue with a variation of the present treatment — although he, personally, advised against it as he felt it was putting us both through an unnecessary ordeal; or — he would attempt to operate.

My mother, who knew his reputation, sat up straight at this point and I have no doubt that the light of battle dawned in her eye.

He explained that the chances of success were an unknown quantity. He had performed the operation only twice before — both were polio cases — and it was too early yet to know if the results would reach expectations. It was a delicate procedure in which the live muscle was dissected into two, one half remaining in situ and the other being transplanted across the leg to replace the 'dead' muscle. At worst it would mean that I still would be unable to walk, I would have faced a long and difficult operation unnecessarily and would spend the rest of my life wearing a calliper. At best, there was the hope that the new muscle would grow and take the place of the old one — and I would walk again.

My mother barely needed to draw breath before making her decision. Of *course* I must be given the chance. If failure would leave me no worse off than I was at present, then what had we to lose?

He stopped her before she had really finished speaking.

'Perhaps I've made it sound too simple a choice. There is another — though rather more remote — alternative result. It could happen that the function of the healthy muscle will be impaired also. It is even possible that, at worst, we might have to amputate the leg at the knee.'

My mother blanched, but remained steadfast. Would having to be fitted with an artificial limb be any worse than wearing a leg-iron? It might be an advantage.

'Very well.' He nodded, with obvious approval. 'But it's not all going to be plain sailing, you know. If you think this last year or so has been time-consuming, you haven't experienced anything yet. The post-operative period will be taxing beyond anything. There will be constant trips to the hospital, exercise sessions at home three or four times a day, special baths — and she must have plenty of outings: lots of fresh air to build her up

generally and to combat the depression that's bound to follow.
You'll really have to work at it — do you think you can do it?'

My mother halted for barely a second before she assured him
that she could.

'You have a family to look after, too,' he reminded her, 'and
you're not what I should call a robust woman. I don't want to
discourage you; I simply want you to realise what you're taking
on.' He added kindly: 'I'm afraid I can't allow you time to think
it over — you will have to make the decision immediately. I feel
it's vital to get on with it right away.'

'Then do so,' my mother said unswervingly. She was the only
one of three mothers, interviewed by him that morning, who
accepted the challenge.

I had two operations and a long stay in hospital. The after-
care was as gruelling as my surgeon had indicated and there
were many setbacks, disappointments and some black periods
when it seemed that I would never be free of hospitals. But
eventually I took those first few steps unaided; I graduated to a
surgical boot and then to specially built-up footwear. It took
three years all told, to the day when I went into a shop and was
able to choose my first pair of ordinary shoes.

My mother — who, years before I was born, had developed
tuberculosis and been given only six months to live — survived
the ordeal undaunted. Despite all the setbacks she was determined that, whatever anyone else said, I would walk again. In
the end she won through.

*   *   *

All this went through my mind on that evening when I faced my
own future and that of our younger daughter — once again the
baby of the family and with brothers and a sister who were full
of love for her.

If my mother could do it, so could I. And surely I owed her
some kind of acknowledgement?

I felt her presence very closely beside me that night and was
conscious of a curious strength flowing through me.

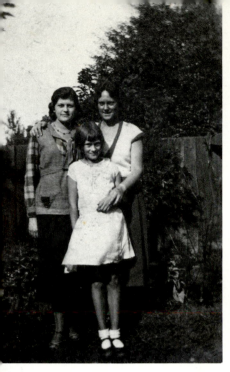

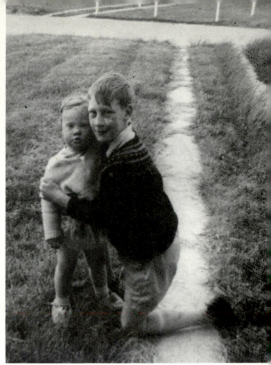

Above left: The author with her two elder sisters, just before contracting polio.

Above right: Cathy, aged 3½, with her brother Michael.

Below: Cathy with Michael and big brother Christopher.

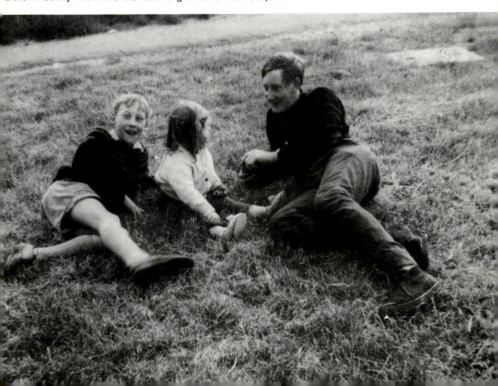

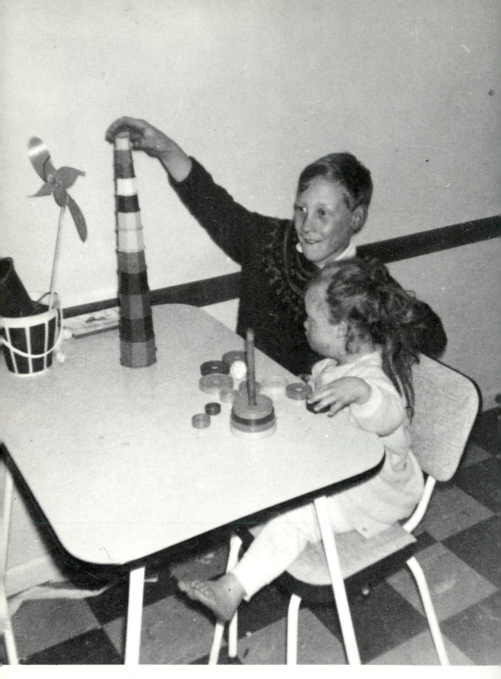

Michael teaching Cathy (aged 4½) with the 'pile-ups'.

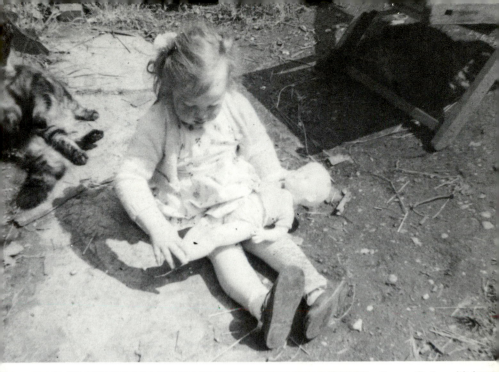

Above: Cathy with her
doll and attendant cat.

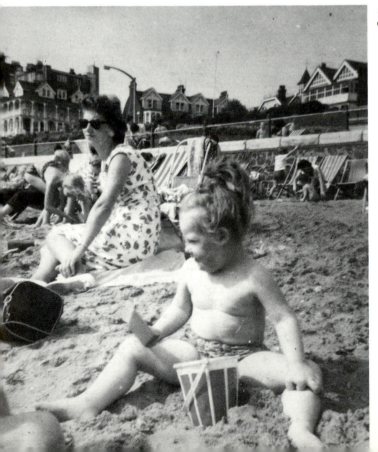

Left: On the beach,
aged 4.

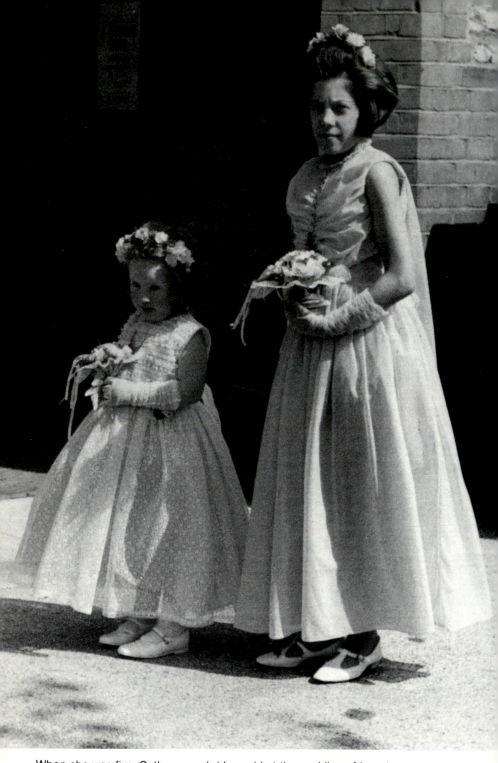

When she was five, Cathy was a bridesmaid at the wedding of her sister, Anthea.

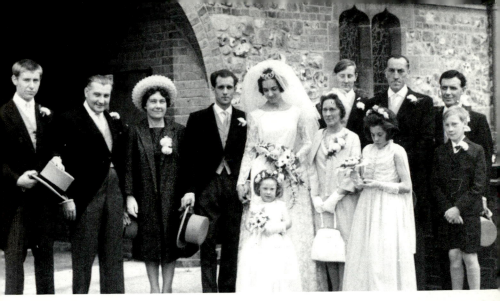

Family wedding group. Cathy stands proudly in front of the bride, while the author is on the bride's left.

A reading lesson. The author is on Cathy's right.

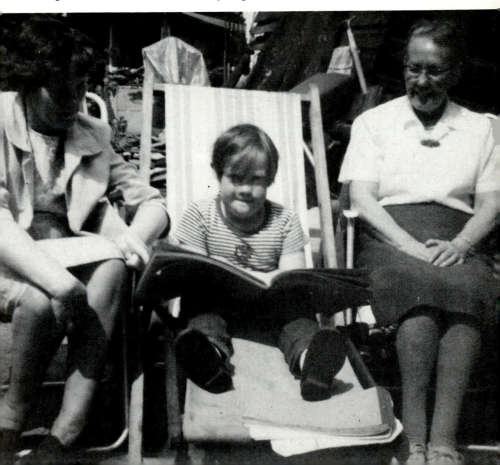

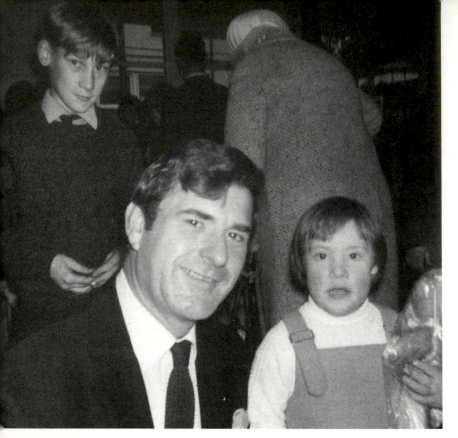

Film star Leon Greene with Michael and Cathy.

Percussion band at Lancaster School. Cathy, aged 7, is on the right of the piano.

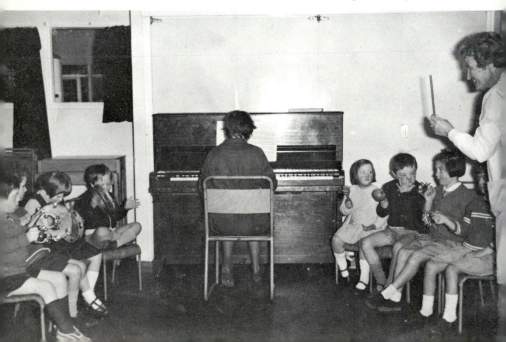

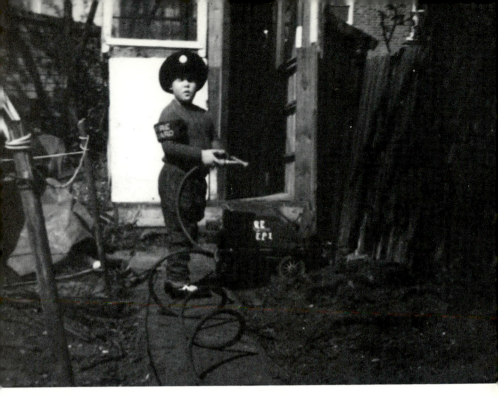

Playing fireman in the garden at home.

Aged 9, with nephew David at Butlin's.

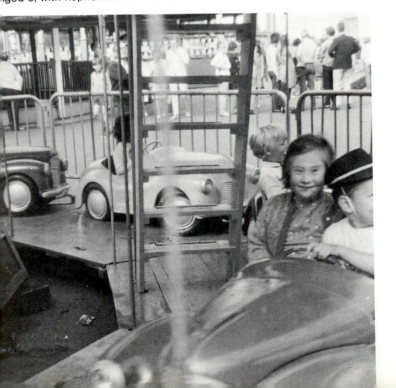

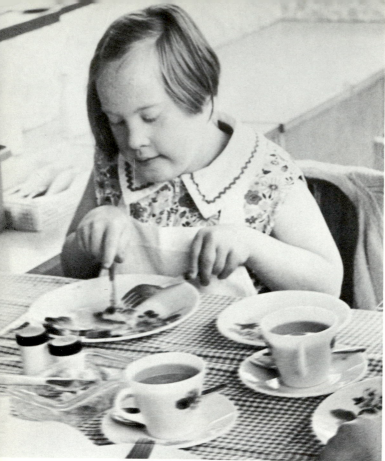

Cooking and eating breakfast at Lancaster School.

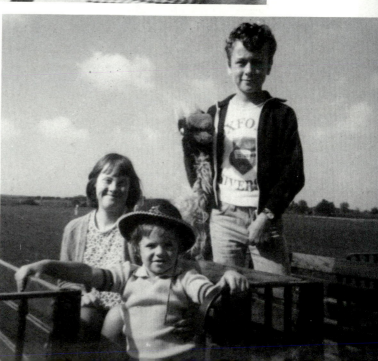

On holiday with David and a young friend.

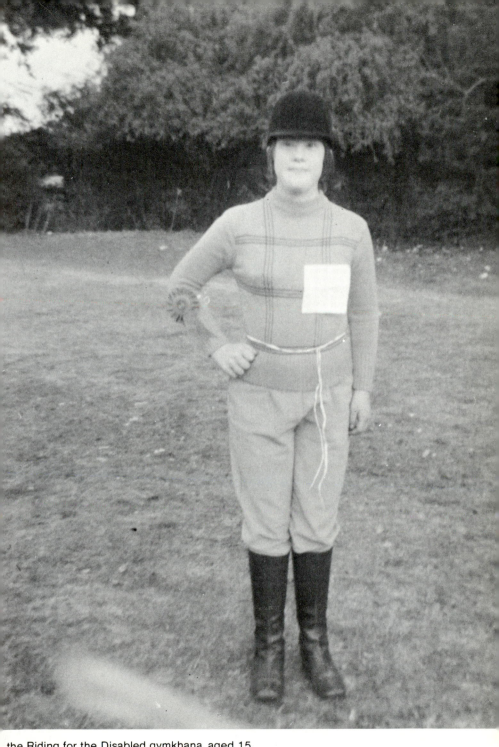

the Riding for the Disabled gymkhana, aged 15.

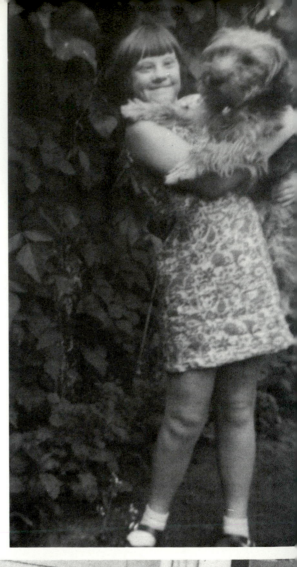

With the much loved SP.

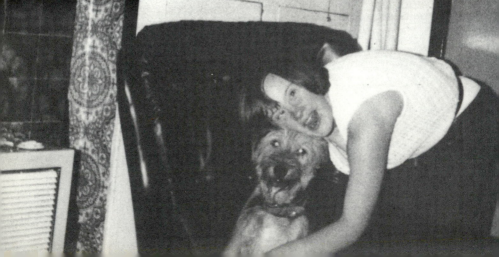

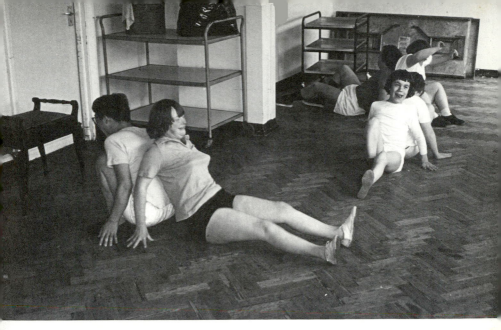

Taking part in PE at Lancaster School.

On holiday in Keswick. Cathy, aged 18, is on the extreme right.

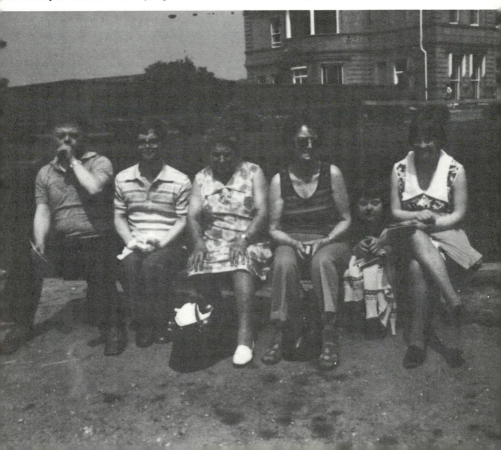

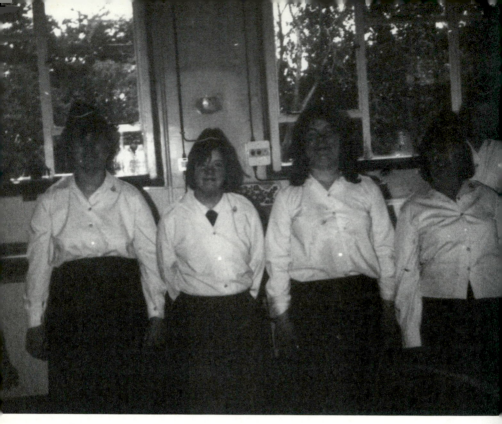

Above: The Handicapped Rangers. Cathy is second on the left.

Below left: On holiday in Devon.

Below right: With the author on the Isle of Wight, 1982.

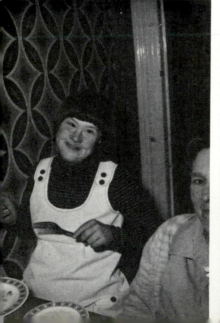

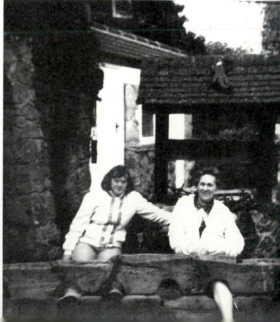

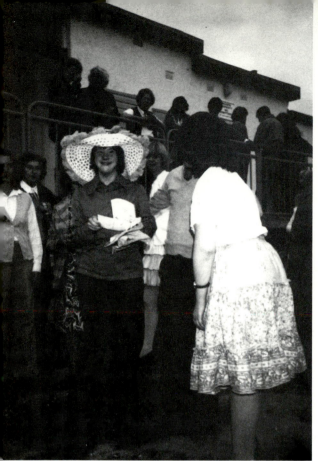

Cathy's twenty-first birthday beach barbecue.

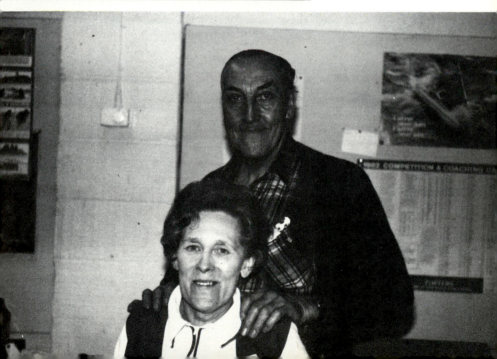

The author and husband Don. 1982.

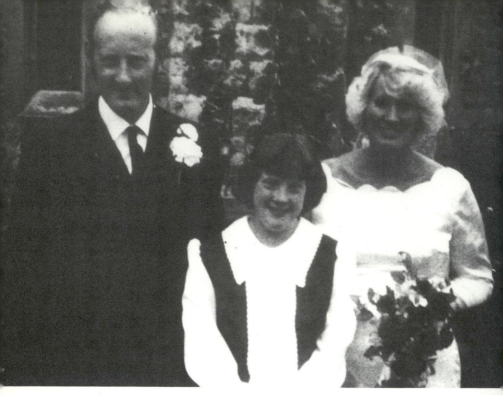

Cathy, aged 21, at the wedding of her brother Christopher.

On a Maybrook camping holiday in France, 1983.

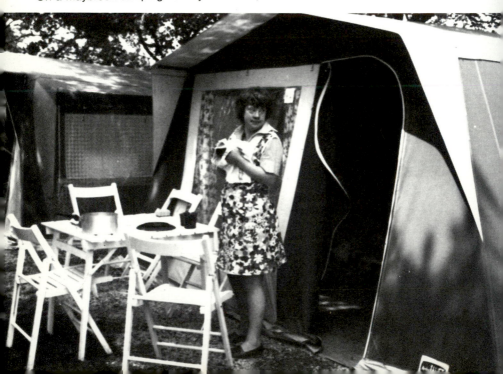

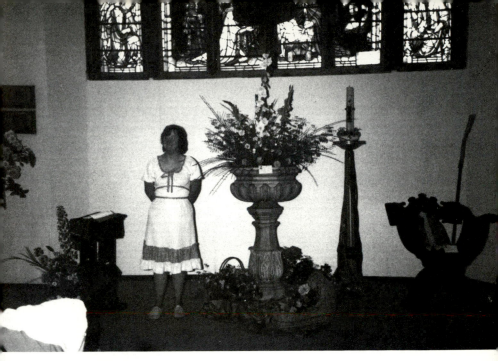

the Church Flower Festival, 1984.

e Duke of Edinburgh's Award ceremony at County Hall, Chelmsford. Cathy, aged 23, ceives her Gold Award from Robert Heron. (Photo: David Mansell)

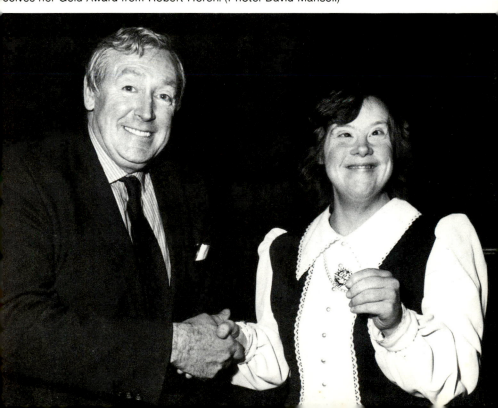

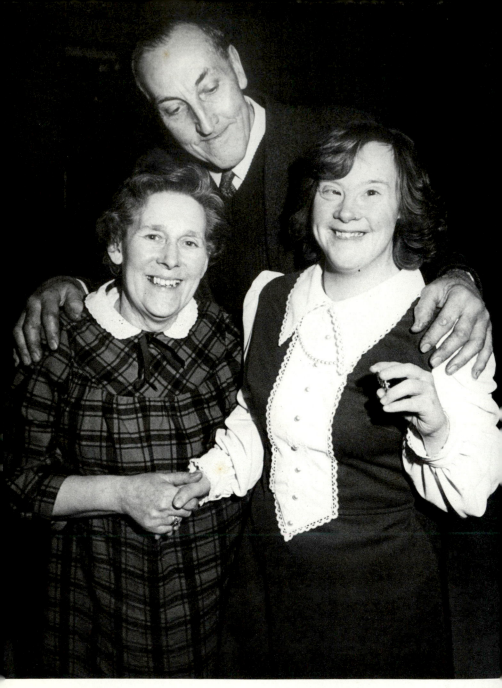

Cathy and her parents after the ceremony. (Photo: David Mansell)

Perhaps everything the books said was true and my child never *would* be capable of living a normal life; but I was not going to give in without a fight. It would be easy to take the line of least resistance and accept the burden without question. I know my mother would never have done this.

So why should I?

Chapter 3

I had to sit down and think about it for quite a long while. I had no knowledge of how to train a mentally handicapped child — but then how many people did know?

The so-called experts seemed to concentrate solely on stressing the difficulties to parents, pointing out what the child could not, and never would, do. No one seemed to be interested in working out a training scheme for developing what he or she *could* do. At least, if anyone had, why had they not written a book about it or publicised it in any way?

The only thing to do, it seemed to me, was to work out a system of my own. After all, it had paid off so far. Without realising that my child was mentally handicapped I had managed to carry out all the basic training that I had given my other children. I had considered that she was simply a little slow to learn.

By letting her grip my fingers while I carefully raised and lowered her, I had finally taught her to sit up on her own. These exercises were interspersed with gentle massage and a certain amount of stimulation by moving her limbs rhythmically while I sang to her. Of course, once she could sit up on her own a whole range of new experiences opened up to her. She could now take an interest in what was going on in the world about her and was able to reach out and grasp the toys and other articles that I placed nearby. These she could examine at her leisure by touch, taste and sight and even by hearing, if the object happened to squeak or rattle.

Even in her 'lying-down' days, I had hung brightly-coloured objects — frequently changed — in her line of vision, and if they turned and moved in the air, so much the better.

The next stage in development came about with learning to

crawl. She managed to turn herself on to her tummy one day and after we had perfected this movement, I noticed that she was trying hard to push herself up on to her knees. We spent some days helping her to achieve this, but once there and firmly established in place, with no flopping, she seemed uncertain as to where to go next.

I found the answer eventually. The trick was to place a favourite joy just out of reach, but well within her vision-range. Carefully, I moved each knee forward in turn, making sure that she remained properly balanced, until she was able to stretch out and pick up the toy. Her joy and triumph then were overwhelming. Repeating this method at intervals, with plenty of rest-time in between, paid off after a few days and she suddenly found she could carry out the manoeuvre without any help from me.

I used the 'toy out of reach' method again, by suspending one of her favourites just above her head. She would reach upwards, until able to touch it, stretching her arms up high, thus further stimulating those floppy muscles.

Since these exercises had been so successful in her earlier training, we decided to continue in the same way. Once she had reached the stage of pulling herself up into a standing position, we taught her to walk by the simple process of two of us holding her by the hands while a third member of the family encouraged her to place one foot in front of the other. Praise, gentle encouragement and plenty of rewards in the shape of hugs and kisses, did the rest.

The answer, it seemed to me, was never to force the pace but to break down the action to be mastered into a series of stages and then to take these one at a time, until each step in turn was perfected. Never to hurry, never to rush at it or become despondent when she did not respond. There was always another day for trying and her visible joy and obvious sense of achievement when she did succeed were well worth waiting for.

Nursery rhymes and songs are absolutely invaluable, to my mind, when undertaking a baby's early training. I think it is very sad that these days mothers don't seem to sing them to their babies. A recent survey showed that about 80 per cent of children tested in junior schools had never heard of most of the traditional rhymes.

For my own part, I found 'This Little Piggy went to Market', 'Pat-a-Cake, Pat-a-Cake', 'Round and Round the Garden' and many others absolutely perfect for teaching all my children when young, and Cathy was no exception. Accompanied by suitable actions, these songs were great training-material and soon she was able to carry out the hand movements on her own. Games of 'Peek-a-Boo' followed, and of learning to wave 'Bye-bye' and blow kisses.

Toilet-training and learning to hold a cup, to drink and feed herself from a spoon had all been carried out according to normal specifications. Again, I had not known she was handicapped but simply recognised that she was slow in her reactions and would obviously take a little longer to learn things than my other children. I used no special methods, just let her take her own time.

From quite early on, we had tried to help her by buying toys that, as well as proving amusing, would also be educational in some way. Brightly coloured bricks and 'pile-ups' and varied plastic shapes which had to be posted into the right holes in a kind of pillar-box had turned out to be extremely useful as well as popular.

The games department was Michael's particular province and he invented some ingenious variations, which they played for hours. Clumsy at first, Cathy's fingers soon became more practised in the art of building towers that did not immediately fall down. The shaped pieces she found more difficult to manipulate but, showing endless patience, Michael would guide her hand until she could manage to complete the operation successfully. Apart from anything else, these exercises in control helped tremendously to build up her self-confidence.

So we progressed, slowly but consistently, for the first four years of her life.

*   *   *

The Health Visitor was making one of her six-monthly visits. All children under school-age received these in our part of the world, in those far-off days when the Health Service was not suffering constantly from 'cuts'.

She looked decidedly uncomfortable, I thought, and seemed to be struggling with a painful mixture of embarrassment and pity.

'You do realise,' she emphasised, 'that she'll never really *do* anything?'

'What exactly do you mean by that?' My voice sounded like a stranger's, icily polite.

'Well, she'll perhaps go to a Training Centre — something like that, anyway.'

I had never heard of such places, and said so.

'They are Day Centres where children like — like *that* are taken,' she explained awkwardly.

It sounded to me like a cross between a prison camp and a juvenile detention centre.

Translating the expression on my face correctly, she went on quickly: 'They are excellent places. The children are very happy there. They are given a certain amount of basic training and — well, after all, even if they don't learn much it does give the mother a break — allows her to forget about the child for a few hours.'

I knew that at any moment I was going to say something I should probably regret. With difficulty I controlled myself and asked politely: 'What do you call basic training?'

'Oh, things like learning to feed themselves —'

'We've already taught her to do that.'

'And to sit at a table in her own chair.'

'She's been doing that for some time.'

'Well — they try to give them a little toilet-training. Not that one should be too hopeful,' she added hastily. 'After all, one can't really expect —'

'I've toilet-trained her in the same way as I did my other children,' I told her patiently. 'She's been out of nappies for ages — at least in the day-time. We're persevering with the nights and she doesn't have many accidents now.'

'But that's virtually impossible.' She regarded me disapprovingly, purse-lipped, obviously quite certain that I was lying — probably in desperation, because I wanted her to think well of my child.

I drew Cathy to my side and lifted up her dress to show off her frilly panties, unencumbered with nappies.

'I think you're taking rather unnecessary risks,' the HV admonished somewhat severely. 'You really can't expect her to know —'

'But she *does* know,' I argued. 'And she's so proud of her pretty pants that she wouldn't do anything to spoil them.'

As though she understood and appreciated our differences — although it was probably the phrase 'pretty pants' that did the trick — my daughter trotted out of the room and returned with her potty, which she presented to me. I sat her down on it and she performed beautifully. I could have hugged her.

The HV stared.

'Well, all I can say is, you've been very lucky.'

Not lucky, I wanted to tell her, just prepared to do something about it.

In the absence of any professional help, we had continued to work out our own training system. My other children had all learned to speak fluently at a very early age, my method having been to talk a great deal to *them*. I didn't see why it should not work just as well for Cathy.

She obviously found enunciation difficult (Down's children have small mouths and extra-long tongues) and I was very careful to form the words correctly, letting her see the particular movement of lips, teeth and tongue. Once she had grasped the idea, I set out to build up a good vocabulary and at the same time emphasise the sense of the words, so that they had some meaning for her.

I let her help me about the house as much as possible and our conversation would go something like this:

'Now we'll make the bed. Which sheets shall we have — the blue ones? Now, you hold this sheet for me and I'll take *this* sheet and put it on the bed. Now we'll tuck it in. Isn't it a pretty blue? It's just like your dress, isn't it? Your dress is blue, too — and my slippers are blue, do you see? Now, where is your sheet? Is that blue, too? Yes, it is, isn't it? Put that sheet on top of the other one — now we have two blue sheets, haven't we? They look very nice in this room, because there are lots of other blue things. Do you see the blue flowers on the curtains? And the little mat here — that's blue, too.'

Usually at this point she would have cottoned on sufficiently well to point to one or two other things and say: 'B'oo.'

'B-l-ue,' I would enunciate clearly, exaggerating the movement of lips and tongue. After one or two attempts, she usually managed to get it right.

In this way quite a valuable lesson had been learned. She could recognise the colour blue and name it aloud, had learned a new word — 'sheet' — and seen how a bed was made. Although it took much longer to perform the household tasks, the work was carried out somehow and it meant that Cathy was learning all the time.

This method was adopted by other members of the household, too, when engaged in any kind of activity that Cathy could watch and enjoy — although I must admit that those not involved usually retreated to a safe distance or sat with fingers in ears, since listening to this repetitive flow of words (strongly reminiscent of *Reading, Book I: language* or *First Year French*) could be extremely tedious and even likely, when prolonged, to send one screaming up the walls!

Nevertheless, the system paid off and is to be highly recommended.

We also ventured into the realms of counting, chanting: 'One, two, three!' every time we went up and down the stairs or set the places at table. Cathy soon learned to say the numbers up to ten, but all young children find it difficult to grasp the real *meaning* of the words and it is often some time before they can relate them to the actual numbers of certain objects.

After trying in every way to convey to her what different amounts meant, I was overjoyed one day when she pointed to a couple of apples lying on a dish and said: 'Two!'

Just to make sure, I added another apple to the others. She hesitated for a moment, then asked tentatively: 'Three?'

'Yes, three!' I agreed and she laughed delightedly. It had taken some time to sink in, but from then onwards I could ask her to bring me two spoons or three plates and I knew she would understand what I wanted.

*　　*　　*

The HV left us finally, promising me that she would follow up the matter of the Training Centre. I was quite prepared to hear no more, but she was evidently anxious to 'free' me from the burden of my daughter and I had a letter only a week or so later, asking me to take Cathy to the Health Centre for assessment.

I made a few enquiries and discovered that a kind of IQ test would be carried out to establish the extent of her handicap. (Apparently, even the local Training Centre drew the line at a truly impossible case.)

We arrived early at the Health Centre, which was a somewhat dismal building — it had once been the old hospital and was rather grim and forbidding-looking.

After a long wait, we were shown into one of the smaller rooms and I was introduced to the woman who was to be Cathy's Assessor.

'It will take some time,' she told me. 'Perhaps you'd like to go and do some shopping and come back in about an hour.'

It was more a command than a suggestion, although issued in the nicest possible way. I wasn't worried about leaving Cathy to the mercies of a stranger; we had so many friends and acquaintances visiting the house that new faces didn't worry her at all. She was, in fact, already casting an interested eye in the direction of some brightly-coloured plastic shapes which were presumably part of the test equipment.

I said goodbye and left her. When I returned, she was still closeted in the little room. A passing official told me that I might as well go in, so I knocked and did so.

The Assessor looked up and smiled encouragingly.

'We've nearly finished, mother. Sit down.'

I took a seat at the table and watched with interest. Without appearing to do so, I cast a quick eye over the paper in front of the examiner. There were rows of crosses in what appeared to be the answers column — but only one or two ticks. I was conscious of a hollow, sinking feeling. Had she really done so badly? Or was I just misconstruing the results?

'We're matching words to pictures,' the Assessor explained. Then, to Cathy: 'Look at the pictures, dear. Can you tell me their names?' She pointed. 'What is this? Do you know?' She indicated an illustration of a girl in a colourful Fair Isle jacket.

'Woo-ee,' said Cathy, smiling brightly.

'What, dear?'

'Woo-ee.'

'No. That's a picture of a girl.' Another cross was added to the answer-list.

I knew I really should not chime in, but — interfering mum or not — I just could not let this pass.

'She got it right,' I said. 'She's saying "woolly". It's her name for a cardigan.'

'Oh.' She looked doubtful. 'Are you sure about that?'

'Try her,' I suggested.

'Look at the picture again, dear. Can you see a woolly?'

'Yes.' Cathy's face broke into a bright smile and she stabbed a small finger at the picture. 'Woo-ee!'

The cross was changed to a tick.

The next picture was of a circus elephant.

'Pippy!' Cathy shouted delightedly.

'What was that, dear? Do you know what is in the picture?'

'Pippy!' Happily repeated.

Another cross went on the paper.

'I hate to interrupt,' I broke in quickly, 'but she's right again. It's Pippy the Elephant; she watches him on television.'

The woman looked doubtful. She had obviously never heard of the character.

'It's natural that you should want her to do well,' she said in an understanding tone, with a decided undercurrent of 'oh, these wretched mothers'. 'She certainly seems to be able to *say* a number of words, but she obviously doesn't understand their meaning; she can't relate them to the pictures at all.'

'What do you mean, exactly?' I queried.

'Well, for instance —' She drew out a sheet of paper covered with pictures of animals. 'She doesn't give the right names for these, although she is actually using proper words. This often happens — mentally handicapped children repeat things just as a budgie might, but the words have no real meaning for them.'

'Could you give me an example?'

'Well, let me see.' She consulted her notes. 'The picture of the dog was recognised as "socks" and the cat was taken to be a "teddy" — a teddy bear, I suppose she means.'

'No!' I had to protest, whether she liked it or not. 'We have a cat whose name is Teddi and our friends have a dog called Sox.'

Either she didn't believe me or she felt that I had interfered enough. The papers were hastily gathered together and the Assessor rose.

'Well, I think we have enough to go on. Don't be too depressed about it — her manual dexterity was quite good, anyway. Thank you for bringing her in.'

We were ushered out of the place. I felt extremely unsatisfied about the whole business. How could a complete stranger expect to get into a small child's mind? Even a normal child of five sometimes had difficulty in pronouncing words correctly and surely lots of children had pet names for things — family names, which were 'in' jokes, such as always calling your hot-water bottle 'Henry' or referring to tapioca as 'stodge'. Wouldn't it be much better to allow one of the parents to act as interpreter? Or perhaps that would merely be regarded by the experts as an intrusion. Maybe they were right and I *was* just an 'interfering mum'.

The results did not surprise me when they came. It was the same old cry: 'Your child has been found to be ineducable.'

It did not shake my determination one iota — rather the reverse. We continued with our training methods. At least

Michael's games with the build-up bricks and play-shapes had paid off, which was a terrific boost for him. Because of them Cathy had scored high marks for 'manual dexterity' and 'hand and eye co-ordination'.

There was a long interval before we heard any more, but finally I was invited to go and inspect the Junior Training Centre.

I do not quite know what I expected to find, but I was certainly pleasantly surprised. The main building had originally been a large private house and then converted into a nursing-home; it was shut away from the public gaze behind high walls. I, for one, had certainly not realised it was there at all.

From the outside the house did not look too formidable: it was neither forbidding nor inviting, just blandly neutral. Once one walked through the main building and out at the back, however, there was a different atmosphere altogether. Bright, sunny pre-fabricated 'classrooms' had been erected in what had once been the garden. There was a large concreted play-area, a sand pit and lots of grass. It gave the impression of being a rather nice, small private school. The classrooms, however, were not furnished with desks but with small tables, low chairs and the occasional wheelchair. There were bright pictures on the walls and lots of colourful toys lying around.

The children looked very happy and were indulging in various simple forms of play. I had been asked to bring Cathy with me and we were taken on a grand tour, finally finishing up in the classroom which would be hers if she were accepted.

The teacher was a warm, motherly-looking woman. (I later found out that she had a Down's son of her own.) She introduced us to the children and was delighted when Cathy repeated some of their names.

'She's a bright little button, isn't she?' she laughed.

'Button!' said Cathy delightedly and pointed to one on the front of her dress.

'Well! that *is* promising!' She smiled at me. 'You've obviously made a very good start with her. Let's hope there'll be a vacancy here soon; then we'll see how much we can teach her.'

It was the first really encouraging thing that anyone had ever said to me.

*   *   *

It was some time before we had any further communication from the authorities.

At last the expected letter came, offering us a place in the Junior Training Centre. Cathy was by then almost six years old; but we were only too pleased to think that she had had to wait no longer, as we had heard that many of the children were unable to find a place until they were at least seven or eight.

Nowadays, things have improved greatly. The old term 'Training Centre' has been abolished and — in the Southend District, at any rate — Down's children are accepted in 'School' at the age of about two-and-a-half, so that their training can begin as early as possible.

Once installed, Cathy settled down very well and seemed to enjoy the day's activities, such as they were. She also appreciated the company of the other children, as she had sadly missed Michael during the hours he himself was away at school.

In the interim, while waiting to hear about a vacancy, I had made two or three more abortive attempts to join in the activities of the local Mentally Handicapped Society. About the only positive thing to come out of this — apart from having actually paid a subscription and having my name and address entered in the rolls — was the fact that we had acquired a dog.

The father of one of Cathy's friends approached me at a meeting and announced brightly: 'I understand that you are going to give a home to our puppy.'

I was somewhat taken aback. We had two cats of our own and one which had adopted us, and I did not think they would take very kindly to the advent of a young and boisterous puppy.

When I explained about this, I was told that SP simply adored cats, as he had been brought up with them.

'SP?' I asked, with curiosity.

'It's short for Surprise Packet. His mother is getting on in years and she's never had a pup before. It came as a complete surprise to us — and to her, too, I believe!'

It seemed that our two small daughters had arranged between them — and apparently in their own language! — for Cathy to be given Clare's dog.

I promised to give the matter my consideration, although actually I had more or less decided against the idea. I knew the boys would love a dog, but it would mean one more pet to look after, to take for walks, to housetrain. I felt I already had my hands full.

However, one wintry night I answered a ring at the door, and there on the snow-banked path were our friends. In their daughter's arms was a tiny bundle, wrapped in a shawl and blinking dismally at the snow-flakes falling into his eyes. He looked so pathetic — straight out of an old-time melodrama, the orphan in the storm — that all I could do was receive him into my own arms and give him a reassuring cuddle. Once that happened, I knew I was beaten!

That was how SP came into our home and into our lives, and what a lovable and loyal pet he turned out to be. Fortunately, he and the cats took to each other at once and Cathy, after a moment's hesitation, because she had never been quite so close to a puppy before, decided that she was going to love him, too. She has worshipped dogs of all kinds ever since.

However, although he plainly adored all of us in his own way, SP definitely decided that he was really Don's dog. It was a case of love at first sight on both sides.

*   *   *

Once Cathy had entered the Junior Training Centre, the pattern of our lives altered slightly and fell into a different routine.

A special coach was provided to transport the children to and from the Centre but it was obviously difficult and time-consuming for it to travel up and down all the individual roads, calling at each appropriate house on the way. Therefore, some children who lived on the main roads were able to be picked up from their own homes, but we — among others — had to walk quite a long way to meet the coach.

When the weather was good we did not mind at all: it was a pleasant walk and we always took SP with us, so he at least benefited from it. On wet days, though, or when it snowed or hailed, it was a different story. There was no shelter of any kind at our pick-up point and we had to wait on a draughty corner, buffeted by the weather, often for as long as half-an-hour. Cathy was the last child on the route to be collected, so of course it meant that each of the other twenty-odd passengers needed to be only a minute or two late for us to bear the brunt of it.

On fine days we did not mind waiting and enlivened the time by singing nursery songs or telling endless stories; Cathy's favourite was the saga of Greedy Freddie — a plot first dreamed up by my father when I was a small child. All our children had adored the Awful Tale of Freddie and his gargantuan appetite, since it involved going into long and intricate descriptions of his various meals and children always love stories about food — one of the secrets of the popularity of the Enid Blyton books!

We were happily singing to ourselves one day, stamping our feet to keep out the cold, when someone passed by on the opposite side of the road, hesitated, then turned back and hovered at the kerb-side as though undecided whether or not to come over.

I hastily stopped singing. Few people passed us in the normal way and those who did were always in a hurry to catch their own trains and buses. At this point I saw the coach arriving and we said our goodbyes, checked that Cathy had everything she needed for the day and I picked up SP, as he always liked to look through the side window to see her safely installed in her place.

I waved the coach out of sight, then turned to find that the dark-haired girl who had watched us from across the road was now standing beside me. We exchanged tentative greetings, then she asked hesitantly: 'Was that your little girl? Does she go to a special school?'

I answered all her questions, feeling certain that it was not just idle curiosity that prompted them. This was confirmed when she told me that she had a two-year-old mongol boy — the third child in their family.

Our experiences were very similar, since Stephen's handicap had not at first been diagnosed — or at any rate, his parents were not informed of any abnormality until some time after his birth. Once she had emerged from the usual traumatic state, she had — like myself — tried to find out something about mongol children and their training — with similarly negative results. She was, at present, endeavouring to contact the local Mentally Handicapped Society, so far without success.

I told her of my own frustrating experiences and we both expressed our dissatisfaction with the lack of help and support available. After all, we were by no means the only new parents of handicapped children. There must surely be some way of contacting others like ourselves, to our mutual advantage? It really only needed a little organisation . . .

I think our eyes must have met at that point and some sort of recognition flashed between us. But we did not, at that time, know each other well enough to follow up the thought.

That was my first meeting with Barbara Crowe, and a momentous occasion it turned out to be. In fact, it triggered off a series of events that were to have their effect on hundreds of parents and children in the years to come. But it needed a third person, who would harness our combined enthusiasm and put it to good use.

Some months later, I had a visit from a member of the Handicapped Society committee. She came along supposedly to remind me of their coming AGM and urged me to make a special effort to attend.

I could not make up my mind whether to be polite but non-committal, or whether it was more honest to be outspoken and voice my many criticisms. After all, she *was* a committee-member and might therefore be partly responsible for the lack of organisation and the totally uninspired meetings.

Over coffee, however, we both let our hair down and I

emphasised my general dissatisfaction and my consequent doubts that I should continue to go to meetings. She, in turn, poured out her own disappointment and disillusion at the way things had been going. What the Society needed, she insisted, was some new blood on the committee and a complete re-organisation of the whole set-up. She mentioned the Crowes. Had I met them? I certainly had. Didn't I think that, being young and enthusiastic, they would make good officer-material? I agreed wholeheartedly. Then wouldn't I please come along to the AGM and second her proposal if she nominated them?

I hesitated. I had already made up my mind not to go that night, since Don would naturally be at the theatre and, so far, I had been unable to find a baby-sitter. My visitor continued to press me, with a kind of desperation. She would send someone to baby-sit for me — wouldn't I go along just for the election of officers, and after that I could leave early?

In the end I agreed to go. I sensed that there was probably going to be a big upheaval at the meeting, that heads would roll and that the Crowes might well need someone — who was also a new parent — to speak up for them. I certainly never dreamed that I would play any other part than a supporting rôle.

However, things turned out quite differently from what I had expected. Several members of the old committee had decided not to stand for re-election. This effectively pruned off some of the dead-wood — although, unfortunately, at least one hard-working and capable person was carried off in the maelstrom, having resigned through sheer disillusionment.

Ken and Barbara Crowe were nominated as replacements and, to my utter astonishment, so was I. Since I did not believe that anyone had particularly noted my presence at meetings, I was even more surprised to find myself elected with a good majority.

A definite current of excited anticipation seemed to run through the hall. After the meeting, as Ken and Barbara and I left for home, I was really touched when a number of people came up to us and said how glad they were to see younger parents with fresh ideas taking up the reins, and how hopeful they now felt about plans for the future.

I feel I must, at this point, digress enough to pay a special tribute to the founder members of the Society. They had achieved a great deal over the years: setting up a sheltered workshop — in the days when there was no Adult Training Centre in the town — and laying the foundations of what had now become the Junior Training Centre.

They had accomplished much by sheer hard work and dogged determination, and without them our children would have been very poorly served. But now most of these good people were growing older and becoming conscious of the ever-increasing burden of having a handicapped child. The ongoing battle with the Local Authority had sapped what little strength and enthusiasm they had and, having laid the important foundations, they were now more than ready to hand on the torch to others.

At the first committee meeting we attended, the remaining members of the Old Guard welcomed us practically with open arms and we were made to feel more like honoured guests than the interlopers we hoped we did not resemble. I had already made up my mind that I would not say too much at this inaugural meeting, since I have a dislike of newcomers who throw their weight about, but we were all encouraged to speak our minds and voice our criticisms, and a useful list of 'do's' and 'don'ts' was collated.

At the end of the evening, I think everyone felt more hopeful and there was no doubt that some very promising ideas had been given an airing.

Next day, a monthly Newsletter was launched and space booked in the local paper for a permanent notice to appear, giving full details of the Society and relevant telephone numbers to ring. No longer would new parents have to search fruitlessly for help.

From such small but important beginnings a new Society was born. It has now become one of the largest and most respected in the country, famous for its pioneering work in the field of mental handicap and with a reputation for introducing new ideas for others to follow.

I can take no personal credit for this satisfying re-birth, although it would be extremely gratifying to my ego to feel that my arrival on the scene had been instrumental in bringing about the changes. It was virtually a matter of luck. Let us just say that the new Executive Committee and subsequent committees, of which I was privileged to be a part, had just the right personality balance, just the perfect chemistry to set things in motion.

Certainly, many important changes came about, one of them being the setting up of parents' counselling groups, which were to prove of great benefit when it came to sharing problems and helpful advice.

Nowadays, too, as soon as a Down's baby is born in this district, the new parents are asked if they would like to see the mother of an older Down's child, who has herself experienced their early shock and distress and is particularly interested in being of help. The answer is nearly always 'yes'. Barbara Crowe or one of her deputies then comes post-haste to visit — usually when the baby is about 48 hours old.

Without exception, new parents have reported their tremendous feeling of relief when hearing the words: 'I know exactly how you feel, for I have lived through this experience myself.'

Another improvement to be made was in the Society's title. At national level it had already been decided that 'The National Society for Mentally Handicapped Children' — later changed to 'The Royal Society for Mentally Handicapped Children and Adults' — was far too much of a mouthful to use in some circumstances. Amended to 'MENCAP', it was far easier to handle and to remember. At local level we became known as Southend MENCAP and found it useful at times to abbreviate the 'Southend-on-Sea' to 'SOS', giving us a rather nice play on words — 'SOS MENCAP' — which was extremely suitable for fund-raising purposes.

*   *   *

Cathy was now seven years old. It was a time of changes; the Superintendent of the Junior Training Centre was leaving and a new Head about to take her place. Consternation reigned; gloomy predictions were bandied about but this was only to be expected, since the retiring Super was greatly loved by the children and both admired and respected by all the parents. Her sympathetic ear and devoted care would be greatly missed — and who could say what kind of person the newcomer might be?

We need not have worried. Peggy Moulder arrived quietly and did not, for a week or two, really make her presence felt. Then things began to happen: suddenly new routines were carefully introduced and we found that our children were actually beginning to learn things.

Sand and water play still remained as part of the day's fun, but now there was a purpose to the activities. How many small jugs of water did it take to fill one large one? And, when full, how many small jugs could the big one actually re-fill? The same number? How exciting! Our children were learning the rudiments of arithmetic.

At home, we were completely staggered one day when Cathy picked up a copy of the local paper and pointed an emphatic finger at one of the headlines on the front page.

'Janet,' she announced firmly, then beamed at us triumphantly as we literally gaped at her. She had, indeed, picked out the name correctly.

'Mum, she can read!' Michael shouted.

But of course, that would have been impossible. Nevertheless, we spread out the pages and asked her if there were any other words she knew. We drew a blank on all the other headlines, but when it came to the 'Births, Marriages and Deaths' columns, she was able to recognise the names Richard and Margaret.

This gave me the clue that I needed: Janet, Margaret and Richard were all in her class at the Centre. Each child had his or her name clearly printed under the appropriate cloakroom peg and also painted on the back of his chair. Somehow Cathy had learned the shapes of the letters and related them to the name of each particular child.

To test her, we wrote down the names of all the children in her class. She recognised nearly all of them.

The next step was to try her with various other words that we thought she might find familiar, such as 'bus stop' and 'corn flakes' from the cereal packet — but to no avail.

'But it does mean she has the ability to understand words and remember them,' I told Michael. We looked at each other in a silent communication that nevertheless spoke volumes. It was a moment full of poignancy, of expectation and tremendous hope.

I reported the discovery to her teacher, who was delighted, although obviously as surprised as we were. She promised she would try to think of some way to use this new-found ability.

As it happened, we did not have to look far or to wait too long. For some time we parents had been pressurising certain MPs about the bleak outlook of our children's future. Training Centres at that time came under the responsibility of the Ministry of Health and had no dealings at all with the Department of Education. Because of this, there was no obligation on the part of the Local Authority to provide any kind of scholastic studies.

The position was quite unfair and took no account of the fact that every child of school age is entitled to some kind of educational training. Many of the children, with only minor handicaps and disabilities other than Down's Syndrome, were quite capable of being taught ordinary lessons in a simplified form and we all felt that they should at least be given the opportunity.

The powers-that-be generally wavered about when faced with this subject (it was not until 1971 that the shift to education was actually made official), but they were finally pushed into a corner and reluctantly agreed that if our children could be shown to be capable of learning, then consideration would be given to the idea.

A great deal of excitement was generated when reading

lessons were introduced into the programme at the Centre. I was fortunate enough to be able to sit in on one of Cathy's early sessions, and soon picked up the rudiments of the system that was being used.

To explain briefly: a set of large cards, each printed with a simple pattern of dots, corresponded to a similar series of patterns printed in a book. The idea was for the child to match up card and book, memorising the 'picture' of the dots if possible.

Once the idea had taken root, a second set of cards, including lines as well as dots, was substituted. Eventually, the line-and-dot patterns were formed into actual letters and words; by now the child had (hopefully) become used to matching up the signs and symbols and, with any luck, would have no difficulty in pairing each 'flashcard' with its partner in the book. At this stage, a picture was added so that the word had some meaning for the reader.

As happens in most schools, the problem was that the specified time allotted to reading lessons did not allow each child more than a very short session at a time. Twenty minutes twice a week was just not long enough, especially when dealing with minds that had a limited capacity for learning and worked at about half the speed of normal thinking.

It was soon quite apparent that Cathy, for instance, needed a much longer lesson. By the time she reached the end of each reading period, she was just beginning to get somewhere; having to wait for three or four days — or perhaps a week — before she could pick up the threads again, meant that she usually had to start from scratch once more and progress was thus painfully slow.

The obvious solution seemed to be to start reading lessons at home. I took careful notes and Michael and I set out to make up our own reading system. We were soon busily engrossed in cutting up mail-order catalogues and old magazines, choosing brightly-coloured pictures of cats, dogs, hats, cups and anything else that had a short and familiar name. These went into big scrap-books and we painted flashcards with the appropriate names on them, using certain colours for certain objects. When all was ready, the lessons began.

Slowly Cathy began to absorb the process and to learn and remember the shape of the words, matching each one up to the appropriate picture with its accompanying name. It was a laborious business to begin with, but we knew it would be worse than useless to try to hurry her. Soon she could go through the book quite quickly, picking up the cards almost without hesitation and with an obvious sense of achievement. When she seemed to be really confident, we discarded the pictures and tested her on the flash-cards alone, getting her to name the words on them. She herself was quite surprised to find that she knew them all!

But so far we had dealt only in proper names or nouns: now came the complicated part. We added some more pages to her book, this time using prepositions and other parts of speech. These were difficult to illustrate but we finally found a way.

A man climbing a ladder, with an arrow drawn alongside and pointing upwards, represented UP; next to him, another man tumbled off the ladder, with a downward-pointing arrow and the word DOWN. We used a hat in a box for IN and a boy going though a door into the garden for OUT. Two pictures of Humpty Dumpty and his wall were ideal for ON and OFF.

When it came to the awkward words like THE, BUT, IT, OF, etc., we realised that it would be almost impossible to link them to pictures; but by now she was beginning to understand that the flash-cards represented actual *words*, so by taking things slowly we were able to teach her the 'shape' of those we could not portray visually and she memorised them one by one.

Adjectives were not so much of a challenge as it was simple to illustrate FAT, THIN, BIG, SMALL, etc; the names of the colours, too — or at any rate the easier ones such as RED, GREEN and BLUE — spoke for themselves.

She now had a vocabulary of about 100 words.

At last we were really getting somewhere. It was time to dispense with the large flash-cards and make her a set of much smaller ones, using all the words she knew. We chose a size that was about the equivalent of the print used in a first reader.

The next few lessons were devoted to putting the words on the cards together to make sentences. As usual, we made this into a kind of game and Cathy obviously enjoyed every minute of it. In fact, we all had fun. She and Michael had a daily session of making up sentences from the stock of cards; gales of laughter usually accompanied the exercise as they invented ludicrous statements such as: 'The fat man has a big pink hat on.'

Although we kept adding new words to the book all the time, I knew that we had now reached the stage where we must try to invent something a little more sophisticated. We must use the sentences and build them into stories, and the stories into a book.

The composition of her first book was somewhat time-consuming but also an excellent mental exercise, since I had to write the stories using only a limited number of words — those which she knew, in fact. I was determined that it was not going to follow the pattern of the boring old readers I had had to learn from and which were still being used in many schools; we did not want pages and pages of 'John has a dog, the dog is big. Jane has a cat, the cat is fat.' These stories should have a plot to them, if possible. I must admit it was one of the most difficult and challenging things I have ever attempted, but I can highly recommend it as an exercise in disciplined writing!

From then on she never looked back. It was some years before I could introduce her to reading phonetically — thus making it easier to decipher new words — but this system of learning the *whole* word, almost photographically, worked very well; even nowadays, when encountering an unknown word or name, she has to be told only once, and from then on it seems to be fixed firmly in her mind.

Of course, reading was not the only thing she had to try to master. We had always felt that to succeed, learning had to be regarded as fun. This was why we tried to make a game of each particular lesson, or sometimes we were able to link it up to some kind of a gimmick.

When Cathy had first been accepted for the Centre, it seemed to me that, to be fair to her teacher, the least we could do was to make sure she could fasten the buttons on her coat and tie her own shoes.

Michael devised an ingenious gadget to help her achieve this. It consisted of a card cut-out in the shape of a waistcoat and coloured brightly. He removed the front facings from an old garment and attached them to the card with buttons on one edge and buttonholes on the other, to correspond. He had already worked out that it is much easier to do up buttons when you can see them in front of you, rather than try to look down your nose and fasten your own. (We had tried encouraging her to stand in front of a mirror while attempting this task, but soon realised that a mirror-image can be extremely confusing, with everything appearing to be the wrong way round.)

The 'waistcoat' worked perfectly and she soon became adept at managing even small, fiddly buttons. A second cut-out — this time in the shape of a boot — was not so successful. She could manage to lace up the eyelet holes quite efficiently, but when it came to tying the actual bow, she was inclined to confuse the two ends of the bootlace and usually ended up with either an ugly knot or a bow that simply fell apart.

We decided not to urge her to keep trying, as failure on her part usually caused great disappointment and often resulted in tears. At intervals, however, we produced the cut-out and encouraged her light-heartedly to have a try — but without much success.

After one such abortive attempt, Michael was suddenly struck with a new idea; discarding the old brown bootlace, he re-threaded the eyelets with two separate cords, one green and one red.

At almost her first attempt Cathy was completely successful. It was so much easier to remember that 'red must be looped, green crossed over and pushed through the hole.' Within days we tried her with the brown bootlace again and she completed the bow without difficulty. I have passed on this idea to a number of parents who were having problems with their

'normal' small children and all have been delighted with the
results!

At this point in her life, Cathy took on a new and important
rôle — that of being an aunt — when our first grandson,
David was born. Anthea had married just before Cathy
entered the Centre. It had been a delightful wedding and
very much an intimate, family affair — since John was the son
of our oldest friends, the link went right back to my own
childhood.

I was greatly touched when John and Anthea insisted that
Cathy must be their bridesmaid. As she was only five years old
— and with a mental age of, possibly, two-and-a-half— I hoped
that she would be able to cope adequately and not let them
down. However, I need not have worried. She carried out her
duties without a single mistake and with all the self-confidence
in the world.

She missed having Anthea at home, of course, but at least she
had now acquired another elder brother! And when David was
born, she was completely enraptured. Although she probably
regarded him at first as a kind of live doll, she was always very
careful in her handling of him and the baby quite obviously
adored her.

Their relationship soon became a very close one and it has
been interesting to see, over the years, how the balance of
responsibility has changed.

When David was a toddler — and even as a small boy — he
followed Cathy about everywhere and became her devoted
slave. She taught him his first words, guided his initial steps,
introduced him to the games she played and would read to him
or sing to him for hours on end. We knew that he could safely be
left in her care, while the household tasks went on around them,
and that she would allow nothing to harm him.

I realised that their relationship had altered when David was
about nine years old and Cathy fifteen. For the first time they
were going to an outside event without Anthea or myself to
accompany them.

David, evidently sensing my feeling of slight trepidation, squeezed my hand reassuringly.

'Don't worry, Nan,' he said. 'I'll look after her.'

And so it has been ever since. Now that he is a teenager and six feet tall, Cathy looks on him very much as another brother. For his part, he does, indeed, always look after her just as he once promised.

Chapter 4

It was not until 1971, when Cathy was ten years old, that mentally handicapped children were drawn into the Education Services and immediately, all over the country, things began to improve for them. The Junior Training Centre was renamed Lancaster School and an all-round educational system was properly introduced.

Cathy still continued with her reading lessons at home and enjoyed them so much that I was forced to curb her enthusiasm at times in case she became over-tired. I suppose I erred on the side of caution, for we are all bookworms in our family and undoubtedly we look upon reading as a form of relaxation.

When she was first beginning to recognise words, I remember her teacher warning me gently: 'She's made a good beginning but don't expect her to get beyond "cat" and "dog".'

I *did* expect it, for I had heard Jill, an older Down's girl, reading aloud. Jill had previously attended a school for slow learners and had also had a great deal of encouragement at home. Hearing her read a simple story from a Ladybird book sent my hopes soaring and helped me not to waver when, feeling tired, I was tempted to skimp that day's lesson or even to cancel it altogether.

My hopes have certainly been more than realised. Not only can Cathy read 'cat' and 'dog' but also 'catalogue' and 'dogmatic'! Her grasp of long words is quite astounding and if she does not understand their meaning straight away, she will always be ready to ask. Often *I* am the one who is stumped for an answer. It is surprising to find that, although one is well aware of the actual meaning of a word, it is not always easy to define it clearly to someone else!

I think part of the reason for Cathy's extensive vocabulary is that, right from those early days, we always made a practice of bed-time reading. Unless she happens to be retiring at a very late hour — after a night out at the theatre or some other social occasion, for instance — we still keep up this pleasurable habit. Consequently, over the years, we have graduated from simple fairy stories via Enid Blyton and the classics, to some of the present-day children's and teenagers' books which are well-written and of a very high literary standard — which is more than can be said of many of the modern books written for adults!

Joan Aiken and Penelope Lively are great favourites, as are Nina Bawden and Roald Dahl, among others. Tolkien, of course, is a 'must'. *Black Beauty*, *Jane Eyre* and, naturally, the *Alice* books have been read and re-read countless times. We have bought her cassettes of these and other classics which she can listen to while following the printed text. This all helps to enlarge her vocabulary and I highly recommend the system. Even quite young children can learn to read this way as there are recorded versions of such favourites as the 'Noddy' and 'Pooh' books, Mother Goose Rhymes and all the Beatrix Potters.

Something else that Cathy greatly enjoys and which has proved helpful to her, is having a play-reading session. We each take several parts in the drama and try our best to use a contrasting voice for every one. This sometimes disrupts the performance entirely and brings the play to a sticky end as — particularly when one of us is playing a scene alone in three different voices and the dialogue becomes fast and furious — we collapse into fits of helpless laughter and become completely incoherent!

Needless to say, our family acting tradition had been passed on to our own children and they, when young, spent quite a bit of time putting on plays and shows for their friends' and our own amusement. As they grew older, they were able to take part in the productions of the drama group Donald and I helped to run, and I continued to be involved myself until Cathy was born, when I found that I no longer had enough time to spare. All the same — as might have been expected — as soon as she was old enough to take an interest, Cathy was introduced to the magic world of show business.

Once she had seen her first 'live' show, we made her her own toy theatre, including changes of scenery and characters that were pushed on and off the stage on long wires, in the old traditional way.

At first she was simply an interested onlooker, but it was not long before she wanted to take part herself in the proceedings. Michael and I devised a short pantomime that she would be capable of tackling herself; we chose *Cinderella* because it was one of the stories she knew and loved best. We drew the characters and painted them in bright colours, then recorded the whole script on to the tape recorder — as usual playing several parts each, with appropriate changes of voice!

The incidental music and songs at first set us a problem, since we wanted them to have a full 'orchestral' accompaniment; however, we managed to resolve this difficulty quite easily. When she was about eight years old, we had bought Cathy a toy gramophone; it was quite simple to use, ran on batteries and played small, six-inch records. After a few lessons she learned to operate this herself and would sit entranced for hours playing through her repertoire. Even before she could read properly, she was able to distinguish one record from another, as I had drawn a small symbol on each individual label, as a kind of clue. Thus, *Old King Cole* sported a pipe and a bowl, *Simple Simon* a meat pie, and so on.

We had added to the collection at intervals, and she soon knew all the tunes and words well from having played them so often. As they were so familiar to her, we thought that these would do very well for our pantomime. Interspersed among the dialogue, they added great interest to the production so far as Cathy was concerned, and it was lucky for us that they suited the story of *Cinderella* so well. At least, most of them did! 'Supercallifragilistic', 'I Could Have Danced All Night', 'Some Day my Prince will Come' and 'Whistle While You Work' were absolutely right, although it took a devious mind to introduce such classics as 'Little Brown Jug' and 'Clementine'!

Cathy soon learned the art of pushing the characters on and off the stage, changing the scenes, and so on. Since the whole thing was recorded on one side of a tape, I had simply to start it off for her and then knew that she would be thoroughly entertained for at least half-an-hour, while I could get on with some housework.

This was the first and most popular of several 'productions', but she naturally wanted to see some more 'live' theatre as well. She soon became quite a devotee and is now a regular theatre-goer and enjoys every minute of every show that she sees. We are very fortunate in having two professional theatres within walking distance of where we live, with others only a short car or bus ride away. Added to this, our town has several excellent operatic societies that stage a number of highly spectacular shows each year; there are, too, many local drama groups, producing everything from Shakespeare to Agatha Christie. We are certainly well-served in this respect and I am sure that Cathy has greatly benefited from this kind of stimulation.

As it happens, we have quite a circle of friends and acquaintances in the entertainment world. For one thing, Don worked for many years in our local theatre, whose policy was always to feature guest-stars in the current repertory productions. The Palace Theatre, Westcliff, is well-known in professional circles, being one of the very few truly Edwardian playhouses left in this country. Actors are always very happy to come and perform there.

These warm, friendly people — with very few exceptions — have always taken a great interest in Cathy and in mentally handicapped children generally and shown considerable kindness when it came to offering their help. I would like to pay tribute to them here; we have frequently taken up their generous offers and asked for some personal item which could be auctioned for charity, or arranged a guest appearance at a fête or bazaar.

Occasionally, the response from the public to the appearance of a favourite 'star' has almost proved our undoing! I shall never forget the day when Oliver Reed genially agreed to open a charity fête for us. He arrived early in the day and Anthea spent a diverting morning escorting him round the town, where — surprisingly enough — he managed to remain unrecognised. But, oh, what a different story it was when they arrived at the fête ground, where many thousands of eager fans awaited him!

Ollie had brought with him his younger brother, Simon — at that time his manager, although, now, of course, a television personality in his own right. We had arranged a triumphant procession along the sea-front, ending up at the park where the fête was being staged. Oliver and Simon rode in a jeep, so that they were well on view to the public, and had the Royal Artillery Motor Cycle Display Team as an escort. The procession was led by the Southend Scottish Pipe Band and included dozens of vintage cars, with passengers kitted out in Edwardian costumes.

I should think most of the town turned out to see this glorious sight and the roads were lined thickly with people. A good many of them followed the procession all the way to the fête-ground, where thousands more had already congregated.

I was waiting at the park gates and hopped on to the jeep – losing a shoe in the process, which Oliver gallantly retrieved, with a pithy comment about Cinderella. So far, so good.

The nightmare began shortly afterwards. Once Oliver had descended from the jeep and — having declared the fête 'open' — set out to make a grand tour, all hell broke loose, Thousands of adoring fans surged on to the ground, all with the same intention: to touch their idol if they could, to speak to him if possible, to claim a souvenir in the form of a button or some convenient article of clothing.

I had often seen films and newsreels of the incredible mobbing the Beatles had to face wherever they went, and I can truly say that our own experience came very close to it. Fortunately, Anthea and I were escorted by the fête Chairman and a couple of other stalwart committee men. We all clung desperately together and were swept along with the mob as though by a relentless tide surging in to shore. I don't think our feet actually touched the ground for most of the time! It was a thrilling but utterly terrifying experience.

At last we were able to manoeuvre Oliver to a nearby caravan and, once inside, we literally had to barricade the door against the rampaging hordes. He spent a long time giving autographs and interviews though the side window and then a torrential rain-storm helped to thin out the crowds considerably, although the most devoted fans still remained outside, gazing at the caravan and getting soaked through.

Oliver spent a considerable time with our handicapped children on this occasion and showed great compassion and understanding. I often read in the papers some exaggerated account of his latest exploits and it seems a pity to me that so much time and trouble should be wasted on building up the picture of a 'hell-raiser', simply for publicity purposes. For this is not the real Oliver Reed. He is a gentle, kindly man, generous to a fault and, to my mind, not in the least like his hard-boiled public image.

*   *   *

The fact that well-known public personalities took an interest in our children and publicised the fact in print and on the air, helped tremendously when it came to educating the general public.

In Cathy's early years, not very much was known about mental handicap — certainly the man in the street was kept in ignorance, unless he himself happened to have come up against the problem among family or friends.

The term 'Down's Syndrome' — a gentler and much kinder way of classifying our child's particular disability — had yet to come into common use and Down's children were still known only as 'mongols'. Even among parents this was looked upon almost as a dirty word. I was taken severely to task one day by another mother, for having said in public: 'Of course, our younger daughter is a mongol.'

'How can you use that dreadful word when talking about

your own child?' she asked me accusingly.

'But she *is* a mongol,' I pointed out gently. 'You wouldn't think it shocking if I said she was blind or deaf or asthmatic, would you?'

'That's different,' she mumbled gruffly.

'But why is it different?' I challenged her. 'Your son is a mongol, too. You're not ashamed of him, are you?'

'Well, I certainly wouldn't use *that* word when speaking of him,' she snapped.

'What would you say, then?'

She could not find an answer to that one. It is certainly helpful to parents that now a more attractive term can be used.

It is strange, though, that people should be so frightened of a word. The term 'mentally handicapped' also gives rise to feelings of fear or dread. The general public is inclined to connect the word 'mental' with raving lunacy or drooling idiocy; unfortunately, they are often frightened of or mistrust our children. I think they truly believe that at the drop of a hat they will suddenly start running amok and attacking everyone within arm's reach. I have lost count of the number of times when I and other parents of my acquaintance have been told belligerently: 'All *those* children should be locked safely away.'

Yet all that is really implied by the term 'mental handicap' is an admission that the thought processes have been slowed up or impaired in some way. We are all mentally handicapped to a lesser or greater degree. If we have a blank spot where a certain subject is concerned, or admit to a bad memory, or can't add up figures, then we have a handicap.

I, personally, have tried on numerous occasions to learn shorthand. Although studying languages comes easily to me and I do not have any problems with adding up figures, where shorthand is concerned I am an absolute fool. I have the same difficulty with understanding how mechanical things work; give me a machine to operate and a book of instructions to follow and I totally disintegrate. There is no doubt that in that particular area of thinking I have a definite mental handicap!

Anathema to me, too, are those people who refer to our

daughter as 'one of *those* children'. On the word 'those' their voices will drop half an octave and the phrase is usually spoken in hushed tones, this being accompanied facially by an almost furtive expression, to denote the introduction of an unspeakable subject.

'My poor niece's boy — he's one of *those* children,' they will say, jerking a head in Cathy's direction, their eyes sliding away from her face.

'Oh, you mean he's a mongol?' I carol gaily, with a broad smile. This is one occasion when I don't use the more acceptable 'Down's Syndrome'.

Generally, though, people are kind and even genuinely interested; they really want to learn about the subject. The media — especially television — has helped greatly by discussing mental handicap openly (where once such a thing was carefully swept under the carpet) and really trying to educate the public.

My only criticism of TV programmes to date is that they tend to err on the sad or pessimistic side. While this certainly enlists sympathy on the part of the viewer and is a great booster so far as fund-raising is concerned, it can be totally soul-destroying for new parents. It underlines cruelly the depressing facts that have already — in all probability — been firmly drummed into them.

Television producers always seem to pick on the worst cases, the saddest children — those whose full potential has never been achieved. I have been tempted many times to write to the Director of Programmes suggesting that occasionally we might be shown the other side of the picture. My intention would not be to push my own child into the limelight, but I could supply the names of others who are leading full and happy lives and whose careful training has taught them to be more or less self-sufficient.

Too often, new parents are swamped by a deluge of negative advice from the 'don't expect too much' brigade. How about a little encouragement, for a change?

*   *   *

Needless to say, despite the pessimism of many people and the lack of knowledge on our own part when it came to training, we still continued to impart as much knowledge as we could and to interest Cathy in a wide variety of activities.

At Lancaster School, between the ages of ten and thirteen, she was learning some interesting things: how to clean her teeth correctly, for instance, and the rudiments of personal hygiene. Nature study was another subject that was introduced; in Cathy's class they grew pots of bulbs and crops of mustard-and-cress on pieces of flannel, and they had a family of gerbils to care for and keep clean and fed.

She also learned to sew, beginning with picture cards punched with holes that were large enough for a needleful of wool to be threaded in and out. From these she advanced to simple stitches worked on canvas and eventually graduated to using ordinary material and a reasonably sized needle.

Soon she began to do simple sums and I helped her at home with her number-work, which she seemed to find more difficult to learn than reading — possibly because the end product was only a page full of figures and not an interesting story! Eventually, we went down to the beach and collected some seashells which certainly proved to be useful aids in our lessons. Cathy loved to sort these and lay them out in various patterns; the principle of tens and units suddenly became clear to her when she learned to set them out in precise rows of ten. She soon grasped the idea that there were ten places only allowed in each 'family' and if a new shell were added, one of the others would have to be moved up into the next line. It did not take her long to appreciate that the same thing happened with a column of figures.

She had a lively, enquiring mind at this time and quickly became interested in any new venture we tried to introduce. Working on the same theme of 'work must be fun', I found that jigsaws were very good for stimulation purposes, beginning with thick wooden ones with few pieces which were easy for her to assemble, and working up gradually to more difficult puzzles with more complicated shapes.

Simple board games were also useful, especially those which involved shaking a dice and moving a counter along numbered squares. This helped her with her counting and figure-work and was much more interesting than simply sitting down and doing sums.

We bought her a set of 'rainbow' dominoes, in which similar numbers were tinted in the same colours, so that they were easy to match up. With these she could pick out the appropriate colour first and then recognise and count up the correct number of 'dots'.

It was quite amazing how many interesting things we found in the toy shops. What at first sight seemed to be simply a fun-toy often turned out to be a perfect piece of equipment for educational purposes. Construction-sets, in which plastic shapes could be fitted together to make such things as chairs and tables and wheelbarrows (which could then be used for imaginative play); mosaic pattern-makers; fuzzy felt pictures; gummed paper shapes — all these were absolutely invaluable when it came to practising hand-and-eye co-ordination or stimulating the imagination.

Michael was very good at inventing games that they could both enjoy. Thus they became, in turn, firemen or policemen or intrepid explorers, and these exciting ventures helped to fill in the long days of the school holidays.

Many of these pursuits and experiments in learning were things that we had never imagined she would be able to tackle. In fact, had we accepted the official label of 'ineducable', most of them would never have been attempted.

In his book *Down's Syndrome*, Cliff Cunningham* compares Down's children who had been institutionalised and had received little or no training with those cared for at home, whose parents had attempted to train them to carry out routine tasks. It was clear that those in the latter group not only developed

---

* Cunningham, C. *Down's Syndrome: An Introduction for Parents*, Souvenir Press, 1982.

well and had a wider range of interests and activities, but they were also found to be more emotionally mature.

I found this piece of information of great interest, for it had always been clear to me that as well as teaching Cathy to care for herself, it was important to instil in her emotional independence.

This period of Cathy's development was a very busy time for me. I felt it was important that Michael should have hobbies and interests of his own and was pleased when he joined a choir and the Scouts, the Chess Club at school and other pursuits outside the home.

Since, however, he and Cathy were both at different schools — at opposite ends of the town, of course — there were bound to be times when a clash of dates made things difficult. I remember when they both had 'open' days on the same afternoon and between exactly the same hours. The only way I could manage both was to career across town in a taxi, making hasty repairs to my *toilette* on the way!

I know this kind of thing happens to all parents with children at different schools, but I think the problem is often handled wrongly when one of the children is handicapped. The tendency is either to neglect the handicapped child in favour of the 'normal' sibling or vice versa — which is probably an even worse mistake to make. Fortunately it is a dilemma that lasts for only a while; the end of schooldays brings its own solution.

Chapter 5

I would hate to take all the credit for Cathy's training. We shall, of course, always be grateful for the conscientious and devoted work carried out by the members of staff at Lancaster School.

When compiling the material for this book, I asked if they would not like to enlarge upon some of the areas of training and the lessons that Cathy had learned. The modest reply was that it was 'all part of the job' and no special credit need be given. Despite this assurance, I would still like to record my thanks to everyone concerned.

These were certainly very important years. As Cathy began to mature, our thoughts turned constantly to the future. I think the mistake that many parents of handicapped children make is to put all thought of the years ahead as far out of mind as possible. This is a perfectly natural reaction; the ordeal of considering what will happen when the child grows up — and the dread of coming face-to face with what seems to be a totally bleak outlook — is often too heavy a burden to bear.

There is one question that haunts every parent of a handicapped child: *what will become of him or her when I am no longer here to do the caring?* Because it is unanswerable, the majority prefer to push it resolutely aside each time it infiltrates their thinking.

Although we, too, found the future a painful thing to contemplate, we felt it was better to face up to the problem and try to find a solution, rather than postpone the issue until a later — perhaps much *too* late — date.

It seemed to me that — in the event of Cathy's having to be taken into care — there were several different options to consider. Hospitalisation was one solution; but I had seen a film about life in a ward set aside for mentally handicapped children, and found it totally soul-destroying. These were not children with any kind of physical disability, just those needing some kind of supervision. It seemed to me that, for most of the day, the inmates were kept firmly seated round a long, bare table, their hands clasped on the table-top, so that the staff could see at a glance that no one was getting up to any kind of 'mischief'.

At intervals, they were escorted to the toilet, washed and given regular meals — then it was back to the table again. There were no signs in the ward of any kind of play materials, books or other methods of filling up the long, dull hours of the day.

We parents who went to see the film were utterly shocked that such places could exist in the second half of the twentieth century. One could not blame the staff — they were un-doubtedly overworked and underpaid — but one certainly questioned the total lack of imagination and compassion on the part of those responsible for such a fiendish scheme.

I tried to picture our own child — happy, active and surrounded by love, as she was — doomed to spend the rest of her life in such a place. The idea was totally unacceptable . . . not to be considered for one moment.

The second option seemed to be a residential hostel — in fact I suppose this was really the *only* other option at the time — and this conjured up quite a different picture. Obviously, hostels varied in quality, throughout the country, just as homes for elderly people do. Some were very good — well-run and com-fortable — others seemed to be much too institutionalised. The answer was, obviously, to search until a really good home was found and to instal one's child in it before an emergency actually occurred. Again, this was a positive step forward that one could hardly bear to contemplate, sensible though the idea seemed to be.

We had already been assured by our other children that, if anything happened to us, they would see that Cathy was well cared-for. It was a great comfort to know this, but we were very much against the idea of their actually taking her into their own homes to live. They had — or would have one day — children of their own to care for and we hesitated to add the burden of a handicapped sister. For, in those early days, it was not possible to assess exactly how independent she would become.

But another idea was being broached and even discussed seriously, and that was a system which had been thoroughly tried out in other countries and proved to be most successful: group homes for the handicapped.

The idea was that four or five handicapped persons should live together as a family in an ordinary house. Between them, they should be able to carry out most of the day-to-day routines; that is, one might be capable of house-cleaning and cooking the meals but not really able to shop or work out a budget. Another might understand the handling of money and be competent to go to the shops alone but might not be able to write letters or to do the ironing. Within the group chosen there would be sufficient skills to carry out all the normal domestic routines.

We thought this sounded a wonderful idea, but its success would obviously depend on the capabilities of the handicapped persons involved. It was true that group homes had not yet been established in this country, but we felt sure that it would be simply a matter of time before they became part of the system. The best thing, surely, would be to train our own child to be as independent as possible in the hope that such a home would be the right place for her. Even if she never attained the required standard of efficiency, surely any kind of training would be an advantage to her in the future? Even many of the residential hostels were choosy when it came to accepting certain residents in preference to others.

We did not sketch out vast and elaborate plans but decided to work a step at the time, letting her proceed at her own pace but always aiming as high as possible.

*   *   *

Our first attempts at training followed the pattern that had already been initiated at Lancaster School. For instance, we were greatly interested when Cathy moved up into a more senior class where some kind of domestic science training was obviously included in the time-table.

One corner of the classroom had been set up as a small kitchen with a sink, cooker and suitable working surfaces. Here the children learned to prepare simple dishes; when they had mastered the art of producing edible toast and either boiled or scrambled eggs, they took it in turns to cook breakfast for the coach drivers. This also involved making tea or coffee and learning to set the table properly with the correct knives and forks, a folded napkin and a nicely-arranged vase of flowers.

Some of the parents were distinctly worried when they knew the children were being allowed to use matches to light the gas stove (under strict supervision, of course) and although it was suggested that the lessons should be expanded at home, angry mothers reiterated that in no way would their handicapped child be allowed anywhere near a lighted match. They turned a deaf ear to the argument that almost all small children are fascinated by matches and any ban on their use practically always results in the child experimenting secretly, often with dire results.

Children will almost certainly have to learn to light a match at some time in their lives; surely the very best thing is to show them the correct way to do it and then to supervise their practising until you are sure that they are capable of doing the job properly. I was greatly impressed with the careful way our children lit the gas during their cooking sessions, also pleased to see that hot kettles and pans were handled properly and with respect. Nevertheless, although I passed these observations on, ninety per cent of the parents involved were against such practices and certainly would not have considered ever letting their child near a cooker at home.

We, on the other hand, were happy to carry on with the good work. I made a point of calling Cathy out to the kitchen if she happened to be available when I was cooking anything; I usually explained exactly what I was doing and why; pointed out the various steps taken on the way and, if possible, let her help with the actual preparation. It was not long before she could cope with several simple dishes on her own.

One Saturday morning, we were astounded to be woken up at an early hour and presented with a breakfast tray containing a pot of tea, toast and scrambled eggs — and it was all perfectly edible! Scrambled eggs later became her speciality and she has now taken over the cooking of this particular dish as her results are much better than anyone else's!

The simple rudiments of laundering and ironing came next at school and, again, we were happy to continue the programme at home. Needless to say, I was severely taken to task by many of the other mothers for being 'irresponsible' in allowing her to handle a hot iron. (I have lost count of the many times, over the last fifteen years, this label of 'irresponsibility' has been attached to me!)

It was so rewarding to see the new skills develop and to share in the extreme pleasure Cathy obviously experienced each time she mastered some fresh task.

However, it was less easy to embark upon some aspects of the training. A 'still, small voice' had been niggling away at my subconscious for some time, but I had done my best to ignore it and to push away the alarming ideas it suggested.

Eventually I was forced to accept the fact that the time had come when Cathy would have to learn to go out and about on her own.

This seemed to me to be a very important step to take, although I knew that this particular part of her training would be a traumatic experience for the rest of us, if not for her. However, I kept telling myself that I would have to learn to let go, if I wanted her to have any kind of independence.

Once having made up our minds, our first experiment was to send her alone to Sunday School. (Our church is in the next street, with just one very quiet road to cross.) Although she believed that she was totally on her own, Michael and I were actually following at a safe distance. Once, when she turned to look behind her, we had to scramble madly into a nearby gateway which had conveniently been left open for us!

I had arranged with her Sunday School teacher to be watching out for her at the church end of the journey — particularly as this was where she would cross the road. On the very first occasion her teacher came to the gate to supervise the crossing, but when we were quite convinced that Cathy was well-versed in her kerb-drill and would not attempt to cross even if a car were approaching from quite a distance away, we let her negotiate the road on her own (although she was, in actual fact, still being supervised from the church grounds).

This went on for some months until I was quite satisfied that she could make the journey on her own and without any problems.

The next stage of the game was to teach her to go shopping. We are lucky enough to live very close to a shopping-centre, and all our local shopkeepers knew Cathy well and had taken a great deal of interest in her progress. I used to gen them up beforehand as to exactly what time she would be coming in to shop, so that she would be expected.

As before, I followed at a distance but did not actually enter the shop, simply observing her progress through the shop doorway and making myself scarce before she set off for home. After a week or two I was quite happy to let her walk round on her own — especially as there were no roads to cross — simply taking up my observation post at the corner of the road and making for home as soon as she emerged from the relevant shop, so that I would be in the house when she returned. Fortunately she never appeared to notice how breathless I always seemed to be when I opened the door!

Shopping proved to be a wonderful training-ground for her. In the early days she would hand in a written list with the correct amount of money, so that all she actually had to do was receive the goods, put them in her basket and return home. Later, when she had learned to read simple words, I would make up a shopping-list of items that she could read out for herself. It took quite a bit of ingenuity at times to concoct lists without repeating myself, and how grateful I was for some easy-to-read brand-names; at that time I bought a lot of Daz and Oxo!

Tea was another useful stand-by as she could read out the word 'TEA'; then, when asked, she could always recognise and point out the right packet. Later we were able to progress to harder words and later still I would give her a purseful of money so that she could select a coin of large denomination or a pound note and have the pleasurable experience of receiving change, which she put back into her purse. This, of course, was in the days when one actually *did* get change out of a pound note when doing the shopping!

Nowadays, she makes up her own list, writing it out herself after looking on shelves and in cupboards to see what has to be replenished. We then check with the list I have made of goods I shall be needing during the coming week.

The cost of living having risen, it is more likely to be a ten-pound note that she takes with her, but she always carefully includes a handful of coins of various denominations, so that if the bill comes to an odd number of pence she will offer the required 25p — or whatever the amount might be. She will report this back to me very proudly when returning home: 'It was nine pounds seventeen pence, so I gave her the note and the ten, the five and the two pence.' Sometimes it is just too complicated for her and she has to admit: 'I wasn't sure, so the lady on the till helped me.'

This ease in handling money is largely due, I think, to our game of 'Shops'. As a child I loved to play with what we always called 'the bead box'. This was a large chocolate box, full of all kinds of beads, shells and fancy buttons, inherited from my Grandmother. My sisters and brother had played with it in their turn and added to the contents. They taught me their special games and in rotation the 'beads' were used to make shops, restaurants, fairground stalls with prizes and whatever else we could invent.

I had kept the box and passed it on to my own children, who delighted in playing all the old games and even inventing some new ones. Now it was Cathy's turn and I helped her to lay out shops with the same old 'beads', some of which must by now be nearly 100 years old. There were round brown ones for potatoes, knobbly green ones for cabbages and sprouts, clear glass ones for onions and so on. We bought some toy money to start with but later graduated to the real thing, and after a while she began to get the hang of it. I suppose the training period took longer than it might have done since, just as she was beginning to grasp the essentials, Britain 'went metric' and our lessons had to begin all over again. Fortunately the new system was easier to learn than the old one, but in any case she enjoyed the games so much that it did not really matter, even if she learned very little in the process.

The money side of the shopping still takes her much longer to work out than the actual choosing of goods, which she has mastered very well. She is quite a selective shopper and, if she does not find exactly what she wants, will choose something similar or decide that a different brand or size will do. She can even recognise a good offer when she sees one and if it is something we buy regularly, she will pick up an extra pack 'while it is cheap' and come home delighted with her bargain.

Naturally, we had a few mistakes to begin with, but I don't think she would now, for example, buy a large jumbo size of something we very rarely use, just because a small packet did not happen to be on the shelf.

Shopping has certainly proved to be a splendid training-ground for many things: with her reading, with her writing and spelling — while compiling her own lists — in learning about money and in exercising her mind when making choices or recognising similar brands.

Naturally, the people in our local shops have all got to know her very well, and if she does not appear some time on a Saturday I am bombarded during the week with anxious enquiries. I have to explain that she has been on holiday or that we have had an all-day fête or bazaar to attend. Many of the shop-assistants have told me that Saturdays do not seem the same to them if Cathy does not come in; apparently she really brightens up their day.

Apart from anything else, I feel that the whole thing has been a good exercise in public relations. Many of her friends in the shops had not encountered mental handicap before, except perhaps in the worst possible circumstances. Now they were interested enough to want to find out more and began to ask me questions — tentatively at first, but without hesitation once they knew I was only too ready to give the answers.

Many of them have become helpers at MENCAP events and some have been able to offer consolation and hope when a relative or friend has given birth to a Down's baby.

They often tell me stories about other handicapped children: some sad, some humorous, some incredibly tragic.

The owner of a small corner shop, who has always taken a great interest in Cathy's welfare, commented one day on her sunny nature.

'But I suppose it's because she leads a very full life, isn't it?' she said, and added: 'Of course you are very lucky. She was obviously born very intelligent. I know you have tried to train her but I'm quite sure she would have found her feet anyway.'

I could not really accept that, but felt I could not protest too much without sounding rather big-headed!

'I mean,' she went on, 'there's another lady who comes in here with her mongol daughter and that poor girl can't do *anything*, although she's about Cathy's age. Her mother has to wash and dress her and cut up her food and so on. She can't even speak — she just makes these noises when she wants things.'

I agreed that it was a very sad case.

'Of course,' she added, 'she's not much trouble to look after otherwise. She just stays in her room all day and her mother calls her down when a meal's ready, then back she goes until the next time. You'd hardly know she was in the house, really.'

Good grief! No wonder the poor girl could not talk! It would be interesting to know how many normal children would learn to speak if brought up in similar circumstances.

*   *   *

So now, as a teenager, Cathy was able to go out and about on her own. To any parent considering a similar system to the one we followed, I would issue a strong warning. Crossing busy roads can be a hazardous and nerve-racking business, even for the most quick-thinking among us. For anyone with a handicap, kerb-drill needs to be thoroughly understood and firmly adhered to.

We instilled caution into Cathy from the earliest possible age and trained her always to use a pedestrian crossing if at all possible, and even then to be extra-careful.

Our efforts have certainly paid off and many a time I have groaned inwardly, when in a hurry or heavily-laden with shopping, at having been taken on quite a route-march up the road and down again, so that we might use the 'zebra' rather than simply cross straight over from one side to the other. I have also been firmly held back from stepping out on the pedestrian crossing, because a car was approaching from all of two hundred yards away!

She is quite right, of course; people often *are* knocked down in safe zones by unheeding or absent-minded motorists and I would much rather she erred on the side of caution, than otherwise.

Once she had learned to negotiate the traffic properly, she was evidently visited with a sense of responsibility for those who were not so able. Without any prompting from us, she made a point of helping anyone blind, elderly or infirm to cross the road safely.

The first time this happened, I felt quite emotional; there was an undeniable lump in my throat when I realised that she had now become the helper, the strong one. Yet we had been told constantly that she would have to be assisted across roads herself, probably for the rest of her life . . .

Chapter 6

As she graduated into the senior classes at Lancaster School, Cathy's horizons broadened; she embarked on a variety of new activities and fresh interests, such as beginning to study history and geography in their elementary forms and learning how to carry out domestic duties. The school had moved into larger premises, and this allowed greater scope and room to expand; for instance, two classrooms had been knocked into one and half the space had been converted into a little flatlet, so the pupils could practise bed-making, carpet-sweeping, polishing, etc. This was obviously very good training for the years to come, but unfortunately some of the parents did not approve and stated very vehemently that they had not sent their children to the school to *work*. (One wonders exactly why they *had* sent them!)

One asset, in the new premises, was a large hall with a raised platform, and school plays could now be produced. Their first effort was a very successful version of the ballet *Coppelia*. It was not danced, of course, but the story was mimed to the ballet music and the children obviously got a great deal of fun out of it.

Cathy played the part of the doll, Coppelia, which did not give her very much scope for dramatic acting — since she had to sit absolutely still for the major part of the performance — but it was a good exercise in control, for she was not supposed to blink so much as an eyelash!

Next came a Nativity play. This presented much more of a challenge as she was cast in the rôle of Mary and appeared in nearly every scene. Again it was mimed to a narrated script, although the children also sang carols between the scenes. As part of the project, Cathy's teacher suggested that she write her own version of the Nativity story. This took her quite a long time, but the finished product had a certain charm of its own,

since the suggestion of 'her own version' was taken quite literally and she wrote the story as she herself saw it.

Her teacher was so pleased with the result that she had it
printed into the programme of the play. I here reproduce the
original text, without alteration:

One day Mary was sweeping the floor and dusting, then
she did the washing and hung the clothes on the line and
used the pegs. There was a bright light and an angel
appeared before Mary telling her good News about her
baby who was to be called Jesus.

She went to see Elizabeth when she went to her house
she greeted her by the arms and smiled and they said
'Hullo' to each other.

Elizabeth took her in the house and gave her a chair to
sit on. Then Elizabeth made her a cup of tea and had a cup
herself. They talked for some time before she went home
she picked up her bag from the floor then she went off to see
Joseph. He was working at his work bench when Mary
came in he stopped working and looked at her and smiled.
He told Mary to go to Bethlehem. He took the donkey with
him for Mary to ride so she packed some things for the
journey. Joseph got the donkey ready. They started out,
Mary is tired and Joseph is tired and the donkey is tired
they were very weary when they came to Bethlehem. All
the Inns were booked up. No room in the Inn. At the third
one he took Mary and Joseph to the stable to have her baby
in the manger. When the Angel gave her a baby to hold she
went back to heaven. Mary lay the baby in the manger.

Before the shepherds came with the sheeps they gathered
them in their pens and sat down by the fire to eat and
drink. An Angel appeared before the shepherds they were
afraid of it. The angel told the shepherds about the baby
they thought about it before they went to Bethlehem to see
Jesus. And bowed to him. Then the wise men came on
camels from the east they went into the stable and gave
him presents of gold and frankincense and myrrh and they
went away with the camels . . .

These dramatic performances were seen by only a small and select audience of school governors and teachers. The first time Cathy actually appeared in public before a large audience was in a show devised for a Harvest Supper at our church.

One item was written round the various fruits and vegetables set up in the harvest display in church; they 'came to life' and had humorous verses to declaim about themselves. At the dress rehearsal, the girl who was to have played the lettuce dropped out of the show, because of illness. At first it was decided that, by careful re-writing, her part could be cut out, but a small voice piped up from the body of the hall: 'I know the words.'

Everyone turned round and regarded Cathy with surprise and the producer decided to try her out. She recited the lines quite competently, so he was happy to let her take over.

The next morning — the day of the show — I had to dash out and buy green crêpe paper and then spent hours frantically cutting out strips and gathering them into frills, then stitching them together to make a lettuce costume. I did not have time to worry about whether or not she would be stricken with stage-fright before the performance; after all, she had never actually been asked to speak any lines out loud before. However, all went well and from then onwards Cathy was always included in the church shows — of which there were many, as we had a Vicar who was very keen on acting.

There were other new ventures being planned at this time, one of which was the formation of a Handicapped Guide Company. It took a long while and a great deal of fighting to achieve this particular goal.

We on the MENCAP Executive Committee had striven hard to obtain permission to form the company — with completely negative results. Physically handicapped girls had been accepted into the movement for some years and, indeed, were greatly welcomed into the ranks and even had a special badge they could win for 'fortitude'; the snag with our own girls seemed to be their limited intellectual scope.

The official decision was made, regretfully, on the grounds

that they would not be able to take the Guide Promise, since they would not understand the true meaning of what they were actually undertaking.

I have always maintained that grasping the *exact* meaning was relatively unimportant so long as they kept the rules. This our girls (since their inception) certainly have done — perhaps more steadfastly than many of their 'normal' sisters. I am sure they are unlikely to be disloyal or rebel against God, Queen or Country, and as for helping others — well, no one loves to help more than the handicapped Guides and Rangers of our company. Even the slowest among them delights in being given special tasks to do and will beam with pleasure at the privilege of being allowed to assist anyone.

From this it will be gathered that we did finally manage to obtain permission to run this very special company. This was entirely due to the dogged attitude and utter determination of several local Guide Leaders (one of them Cathy's teacher) who refused to take 'no' for an answer.

Based at Lancaster School, the Guide Company was finally formed in 1978, when Cathy was 17. As the older girls reached maturity, a Ranger Company automatically evolved and is now flourishing, meeting at a local church hall. The girls go to camp every year and spend days out at Guideacres and other sites. We are always very proud of them at the annual Renewal of Promise service, when they parade with all the other guides in the district and are undoubtedly among the smartest of those present.

Cathy enjoys her Ranger activities immensely and has even managed to attain some badges. When she had finished her initial training and passed the preliminary tests, her Leader decided that, rather than enrol her at one of the weekly meetings, it would be nice if her Promise could be made in church during a Sunday service.

This was arranged and everyone turned up in force to support her. It was a very moving moment when she stood at attention, saluted and declared with great fervour that she promised to:

'. . . do my best to do my duty to God,
to serve the Queen and help other
people;
to keep the Guide Law;
to be of service in the Community.'

I was greatly touched to learn afterwards that a good many members of the congregation had been in tears — not because they were thinking with sadness of 'what might have been', but because they were filled with a sense of joy and love, remembering the years of Cathy's growing-up, which had led to this final achievement.

Although Cathy loved her Ranger meetings with the other handicapped girls, her Leader, Marilyn Brown, felt that she would benefit greatly by being attached also to a regular company, whose programme encompassed a greater range of activities than could be undertaken by the less able girls.

Accordingly, she began to attend the meetings of our own church company. Since she was much older than any of the other girls there — and officially over the maximum age for a guide — she was not actually attached to any patrol, but Brenda, the Leader, gave her certain responsibilities and allowed her to act as a kind of Assistant Leader. This seemed to work quite well and, when the day came that Brenda was unable to attend because of illness, Cathy was able to cope on her own with the evening's activities — the guides responding magnificently by following her orders and giving her loyal support.

There is no doubt that this experience of leadership has given her an added maturity and sense of responsibility, which has stood her in good stead at times; we are most grateful to Brenda for having offered her the chance.

Chapter 7

When Cathy was sixteen, we saw no reason why she should not join with the other young people at our church who were due to be confirmed. She seemed to have a good grasp of what the Communion was all about and loved to walk up with everyone else, even if she could receive only a blessing.

Our Vicar at that time (the Rev Ivor Hancock) and I had a talk about it and he was all in favour of the idea, but felt that he would also have to consult the Bishop who would be officiating.

Consent was soon forthcoming and Cathy found another good 'friend' in the Rt Rev Derek Bond, the Bishop of Bradwell. He not only responded with sympathetic understanding and gladly gave his support, but has also shown great interest in her ever since.

No matter how important the occasion, he always manages to find the time for a friendly chat. She calls him 'my' Bishop and eagerly scanned the TV screen on the occasion of the Pope's visit to Canterbury Cathedral to see if she could spot him among the many dignitaries present.

We have explained to her that he is an important person and *she* must not approach *him*, especially when he is surrounded by VIPs. However, she is usually compensated for her acceptance of this rule.

When our current Rector, the Rev Bob White, was licensed, an impressive ceremony took place. A large number of the local clergy had promised to attend, also members of various visiting church choirs and guilds.

'Will *my* Bishop be there?' Cathy asked at once and was delighted to hear that he would, indeed, be performing the ceremony.

On the great day, the many robed figures made up an impressive display and at the end of the service a long procession formed and proceeded up the centre aisle with much pomp and dignity. The Bishop was at the rear of the procession, resplendent in his golden robes and mitre. Many people bent a knee as he passed by, but when he reached Cathy's side he not only returned her broad, welcoming grin but halted the entire proceedings while he gave her a special hug, to which she responded gleefully. Bless him!

Bishops come in all shapes and sizes and some people are inclined to be overwhelmed by their apparent magnificence. Which reminds me of a story — a true one — which I feel is worth re-telling.

Some friends of ours, the organist and leading soprano in a local church choir, had offered to entertain a visiting Bishop — their Vicar having no wife to play hostess for him. They decided to serve him afternoon tea instead of their usual free-for-all family meal; at the appropriate time they escorted the Bishop to a lace-covered table elegantly set with all the traditional English fare: toasted muffins, cucumber sandwiches, plum cake — in fact, the lot.

Their small son was obviously overawed by the whole proceedings. He had seen the Bishop, dressed in all his glory, at the Confirmation service that afternoon. Ever since his arrival at the house, Andrew had regarded him with open-mouthed wonder. Even with a change of clothes, this distinguished man obviously impressed him greatly.

He remained tongue-tied throughout most of the meal and was at last heard to ask his father in a loud stage-whisper: 'Daddy, shall I pass God the biscuits?'

Unconscious humour on the part of children often raises the biggest smile in religious circles. Once Cathy brought home from school a picture that she had drawn of our church, St Alban's. Underneath she had written: 'This is the church I go to. It is called St All-Bran's.'

I was immensely tickled and showed it to Father Ivor. Naturally, he simply loved it — and displayed it at the back of the church, with his written comment underneath: St All-Bran's — for REGULAR churchgoers, of course.'

* * *

In recent times, the question arose of whether it would be possible for Cathy to fill the rôle of sidesman — something she was very anxious to do. She had, in fact, entered her own name on a list designed for members of the congregation who were willing to take on this office.

The Church Council debated the issue and considered what the duties of a sidesman might actually include. These were not too difficult to carry out: handing out the service books and notices when people were arriving, taking up the collection plate, ringing the bell and generally tidying up after the service, making sure that everything was put away in its proper place.

It was finally agreed that as she was quite capable of doing all these things and was now 'of age', she should be allowed to serve.

A six-months' probationary period was suggested and at the end of that time, it was unanimously decided that she filled the rôle more than adequately. Not only was she very conscientious about carrying out her various tasks and always arrived at the church well ahead of time, but her warm personality was considered to be an added asset.

As one of the Councillors put it: 'The most important part of the work is speaking to people as they come in, greeting them with friendliness and a big smile — and who is better at doing that than Cathy?'

Indeed, she is a great example to the rest of us, for surely the hardest, but most important, part of being a Christian is learning to love one's neighbour.

How very difficult it is at times even to *like* X or Y. Cathy, however, genuinely *loves* people. Differences in colour, class, creed or age do not matter at all to her — she believes that everyone is her friend.

This friendliness that she offers to the members of our church

is returned a thousand-fold. The love, support and encouragement that she has received from them has, I am sure, gone a
long way towards helping her to gain self-confidence and to
mature spiritually along the right lines.

*   *   *

From her very earliest Sunday School days, Cathy has always
enjoyed going to church.

As we had done with our other children, while she was still
quite young we tried to give her the firm basis of a religious
training. I have always felt that a certain belief in God's love is
of great comfort to a small child. Thunderstorms, dark houses
and other natural terrors all become less frightening with the
knowledge that 'Someone up there' cares.

I was not at all sure if the major part of my teaching would
sink in or, indeed, how much a mentally handicapped child
could actually grasp and make use of; but I was careful to
explain everything in simple terms, as one would to any very
young child. I felt it was important that she should not only
enjoy the stories I told her but should fully understand that
these events had actually taken place and were part of one long,
continuous story, so that one incident led to another to make up
a significant whole.

Jesus, for instance, had to be introduced to her as a colourful
and interesting personality whose life — right from his most
unusual birth (with all the delightful legendary trimmings) to
his violent death and beyond — was as fascinating a piece
of literature as any favourite fairy story or exciting tale of
adventure.

There are ways and ways of telling stories to children and
even the most familiar nursery tale or the dullest chunk of
history can be given a new twist or made to come alive if
presented in the right way. The characters involved should be
brought to life and fleshed-out with interesting personal details
and flashes of humour, until they become old friends and the
listening child, at the end of the story, begs for 'more'.

By using this method I was able to catch Cathy's interest and whet her appetite for further details; visits to shows such as *Godspell* helped to stimulate her further. We were also lucky enough to get tickets — much in demand — for Alec Mc-Cowan's masterly one-man show: his own interpretation of the Gospel according to St Mark.

From simple Bible-stories we progressed to broader principles, and her response has been staggering.

The family service on Sunday is one of the highlights of her week and she is bitterly disappointed if something prevents her going. Not even hail-stones and knee-high snow are allowed to be deterrents!

Although completely tone-deaf, she sings all the hymns with great vigour, especially those she calls sing-along ones (usually old favourites with a chorus, such as 'Onward Christian Soldiers', or the new charismatic songs, of which she is particularly fond). During these, she will carry out what we call her Malcolm Sargent act. That is, while singing lustily, she also 'conducts' the music with many a professional flourish.

As we sit near the front of the church, visiting preachers are often somewhat non-plussed by her performance, but usually, by the end of the service, they have been won over and make a special point of coming to speak to her afterwards.

There is no doubt she has an incredible faith of her own, and could probably teach us all a lesson. God is very real to her and she firmly believes that He is always on her side.

She will pray very hard for good weather, help in finding a lost article or healing for someone in pain. All receive equal attention and she firmly believes that her wishes will be fulfilled. The strange part is that very rarely is she disappointed. Or perhaps I should not find that strange. After all, we have all been told of 'faith that can move mountains'.

At first I felt anxious, in case some special request would not be dealt with in the way she expected. (I should have had more faith!) Once, when I cautioned her: 'Don't bank on it too much, my love; your prayer might not be answered,' she looked at me in surprise.

Then she repeated something that Father Bob had told her: 'God always *answers* prayers, but sometimes he has to say "no".'

Despite her handicap, she obviously spends time thinking about such things and works out her own conclusions. Once, when we were watching a TV documentary about the loneliness often suffered in old age, she turned to me, puzzled.

'But no one's ever really alone, are they? They always have God with them. Don't they know that?'

I tried to explain that not everyone had the same beliefs, but she found that quite difficult to grasp.

'But why *don't* they? Do they like being unhappy? Couldn't someone tell them? I think God would want them to be friendly.'

This last is an obvious conclusion on her part. She always talks to God in a chummy 'man-to-man' way.

'If you don't mind, God, I'll go on telling you about that tomorrow,' I heard her say once, and she often starts her prayers with, 'God, could I ask you something?'

Sometimes when we have been out and are on our way home, the first few drops of an imminent rain-shower will fall. 'Just a minute, God,' Cathy will say anxiously, peering skyward. 'Could you let it stop just until we get home?' Miraculously, it almost always does.

As we reach the shelter of our front door and the rain really begins to fall, we scramble inside, grateful to have 'just made it'.

Startled passers-by will then cast a wary eye in our direction as we wave a friendly hand and carol in chorus: 'Thanks, God!'

It's all a matter of logic, in Cathy's philosophy. Since she has no enemies on Earth, why should not God be her friend, too?

Chapter 8

'Of course, she'll never be able to *work*, though, will she? I mean — not to do a proper job.'

This is an echo of the old 'she'll never do anything' strain; once we had disproved *that* particular theory, it seemed as though people had to find a further dampener, just in case we were getting too uppity!

Far from being unable to work, Cathy has already established herself in several jobs.

While she was still at Lancaster School, an experiment in Work Experience was attempted. Cathy and one of her friends, Andrew, were released for two — and then three — days a week to go and learn a job at a local toy manufacturing company.

They started off in the packing department, then Andrew was transferred to the workshop, Cathy to the office. When she had mastered the simpler jobs of labelling the boxes and keeping the stock cupboard tidy, her boss discovered that she could read and allowed her to make up some of the orders. Although she could not recognise certain of the words on the order list, she managed to carry out the job without making a mistake by following her usual practice of matching up the 'picture' of the word on the invoice with the corresponding one on the appropriate box.

Their kindly employer was very sympathetic to those in the community who were handicapped and was quite prepared to offer jobs to Cathy and Andrew, as soon as they were quite ready to take them. Although he was not allowed officially to pay them, since they were to all intents and purposes still at school, he would regularly make them up a small wage-packet each, which came out of his own pocket.

We were delighted to think that Cathy might actually be able to hold down a job and that she should be working for such a very kind and understanding man. Unfortunately, before these plans could come to fruition, the firm was bought up by another company and the new proprietor did not wish to have handi-capped people on his staff, so the promised employment never materialised and our two children reverted once more to being just ordinary pupils at a special school.

My own boss had always taken a great interest in Cathy's welfare and shown considerable understanding when it came to regulating my hours to fit in with the routine of taking Cathy to and from the coach.

During some holiday times she had to accompany me to the office, where she occupied a desk of her own, bringing in enough books and pastimes to keep her amused for the afternoon. She simply loved this and looked on 'office hours' as a special treat.

As she grew older, she showed signs of wanting to take part in the actual work going on around her. We gave her a few simple jobs and found that she was quite capable of mailing leaflets, sticking on stamps and even making up packs of advertising material ready for despatching.

Her visits to the office became a regular part of the holiday routine and she obviously enjoyed them greatly. She next mastered the technique of using the photocopier and became adept at collating and stapling sets of pages into booklets.

My employer was astonished at the way she would tackle quite a long task and stick at it doggedly until it was done — despite his constant suggestions that she might like to take a short break — and he eventually made me a most generous offer. If no vacancy occurred for her at Maybrook, the Adult Training Centre, or if I would be happier to have her with me, then he would employ her as an office junior and train her to do such duties as were within her grasp.

I was immensely touched by this suggestion and gave it a great deal of thought. However, when a place was at last found for her at Maybrook, I had already decided that it would be better for her not to be constantly in my company. To achieve true independence, she needed to be away from the home environment for at least a part of each day; added to that, I did not want to deprive her of the companionship of people of her own age.

I am quite certain now that I was right. She had not been at Maybrook for very long when we noticed a change in her. A new maturity was apparent; she was now no longer a child — the baby of the family — but a 'young lady'.

I admit quite honestly that, up to when she was eighteen, I hated the idea of her leaving school and attending an Adult Centre. She was so happy at Lancaster School and it seemed a pity to take her away from the people with whom she had mixed daily for nearly twelve years. But I would impress upon all parents who dread the day when their child must leave special school, the need to remember this: it is vitally important for this break to be made.

In their hearts, many parents never wish their normal children to grow up and break away. They would prefer to keep them slightly dependent for ever, and the day when they finally leave home is something to be faced with dread. All the same, it is a necessary part of life and I think we have all met up with the unfortunate son or daughter still under the thumb of a managing, possessive mother — who is usually rather fond of declaring: 'He (or she) doesn't want any other companion but me.'

So it must be with the handicapped child. That utter dependence on the parent is something which must studiously be avoided, if possible. One should ever be conscious of the future and the thought that Mum or Dad won't always be available. The death of a parent and the consequent shift at short notice to a hostel or other institution is always much more traumatic for the child who has never been allowed to stray too far from Mother's side.

* * *

The transition from Lancaster School (which might be classed as a Training Centre for children) to Maybrook Adult Training Centre, was quite a big step for Cathy to take. Not only would she be on unfamiliar territory and in a work environment rather than a protective school setting, but she would now be a very small fish in a much larger pond.

At school she had finally achieved the coveted position of Head Girl — now she would be the youngest and newest trainee in an Adult Centre; even in small things she would have to adjust to a different routine and learn new rules. At school, for instance, dinner money was paid by the week and handed to the attendant in charge of the coach. At the Centre trainees had to learn to manage their own money and order and pay for their own lunches — a splendid exercise in self-sufficiency. Possibly most important of all were the travelling problems.

Trainees arrived at Maybrook in one of two ways: they were collected and delivered by coach or minibus — just as they had been at school — or they made their own way on foot or by public transport. We were advised very strongly to let Cathy take the latter course straight away. Once she became used to the easier mode of travel, it would be much harder for her to make the transition.

It was like shifting back in time to those earlier days when she first went out alone. We had survived the trauma of that; but could we go through it all again — and this time know that she was facing added hazards? Once more we thought about the future and the unavoidable truth that we would not always be here to accompany her on buses or transport her by car. It did not take us long to decide — obviously there was now one more lesson that she must learn.

The first week had a somewhat nightmarish quality to it. It was almost as though some imp of mischief had decided to torment Cathy — and certainly us! — by submitting her to every kind of difficulty known to bus travellers!

Journeys *to* the Centre were more or less trouble-free, with the exception of one occasion when she was unlucky enough to meet up with a driver/conductor (for these were 'one man operated' buses) who obviously did not like the idea of having a handicapped person to contend with.

Having asked for 'Maybrook Centre', she was then put through a kind of third degree: 'Where's that? — Southchurch Road — oh, yes, but what's the name of the nearest stop? — You don't know? Well, if you don't know where you're going, you'd better get off the bus.'

Maybrook is actually on the main road; it is a few yards only from a bus stop, which lies between two branch roads, neither of which was named on the bus time-tables. The driver knew this very well, I am sure, but was determined to be difficult. Fortunately, a near-neighbour of ours happened to be on the same bus and came to Cathy's rescue. She also reported the matter back to me and to the bus company. Our son-in-law, too, went down to the bus garages and had a word with those in charge. He explained Cathy's difficulties and pointed out that we were doing our best to teach her to be confident when travelling alone. From then onwards, I am happy to say, drivers went out of their way to be helpful. They soon became her 'friends' and on a wet day, many of them would stop right outside the Centre so that she would not have to walk through the rain!

But it was on the homeward journeys that the worst difficulties arose. Almost everything that could possibly go wrong, actually did! On the very first day, she climbed happily aboard, only to be told by the driver that they were travelling to the bus station only, instead of all the way home. This meant — when she got off — crossing the road to a different stop and getting on a second bus.

Next day, the bus she was in broke down *en route* and she had to alight in a strange road at a stop she had never seen before and wait for ten minutes to catch the next bus. Yet another was involved in an accident with a speeding car (luckily with no casualties) and the passengers were kept waiting for nearly half-an-hour before being allowed on their way.

Don had taken a week's leave and, without letting her know he was there, parked just around the corner each afternoon until he had seen Cathy emerge from Maybrook and get on the bus. Then he would drive home ahead of her and wait at a convenient place where he could watch her dismount at the right stop. On the numerous occasions when the bus either did not turn up at all or arrived without her on board, he would make a hasty dash indoors to check if she had somehow beaten him to it, then immediately rush out again to try to find her.

Between us we went through agonies of apprehension and almost decided to give up the whole idea of her travelling alone. However, each time she seemed to cope perfectly well with the emergency and arrived home full of confidence and bursting with the desire to tell us what had happened to the bus. At the end of a week we felt that she had now met up with practically every hazard she was likely to encounter, and must surely be well on the way towards coping efficiently with independent travel.

These experiences, although somewhat harrowing to the rest of us, were all part of the maturing business. I was naturally relieved to know that she was now quite confident about travelling to the Centre — or any other familiar place — alone. I did not, of course, visualise then exactly how far this confidence would one day take her.

*   *   *

In the same way as ordinary schools and colleges, Adult Training Centres vary in quality considerably from place to place.

A great deal depends on the Manager or person in charge, the staff and the attitude of the Local Authority concerned.

Some Centres may include a sheltered workshop where jobs can be taught and carried out under careful supervision. Ideally there should be further education opportunities, facilities for sports and crafts, and all grades of handicap should be catered for.

Maybrook had all these things and Cathy was able to continue with her studies, attending classes for reading and writing and learning how to handle money. She also went swimming and riding and spent some time in the workshop, sampling many different kinds of work to see which one would suit her best.

She settled down very happily and thoroughly enjoyed taking part in the work routine. The boys had an excellently equipped woodwork shop, in which they made some really beautiful things to sell: coffee tables, garden benches, bird houses and various kinds of trellis-work. The girls were mostly on contract work for several outside firms, assembling, packing and labelling a variety of things. Those less able to work had a craft room and other facilities to keep them busy or amused.

Cathy worked on various projects, over a period of time, until she finally found her niche in the domestic department. She became one of a group of trainees whose duties were providing meals for the Centre and also becoming involved in Community Service work by manning coffee bars in two of the local colleges and the Police Canteen. These ventures have proved tremendously successful, both financially and as an exercise in public relations, proving that integration really does pay — in every sense of the word. Cathy is being given an excellent training that includes preparing and serving well-balanced meals and the various domestic duties that accompany this. She is very meticulous in her approach and, when helping me in the kitchen at home, will keep a stern eye on what I am doing, as the work must not be skimped in any way!

She really enjoys the days when it is her turn to work in one of the coffee bars. She is quite confident about dealing with members of the public, who in their turn have been most impressed by the politeness and efficiency of the girls who serve them. Once again, an excellent way of teaching others not to fear or be distressed by young people with a handicap.

*   *   *

When she first started attending the Centre, the trainees were already rehearsing their Christmas pantomime, which was to be *Cinderella*. As she was so keen on acting she was allowed to join the cast, but since all the main parts were already filled, she joined the chorus line. This involved appearing as a Village Girl — the Villagers opened up the show with a lively country dance — a Court Lady in the Ballroom scene and as one of the four 'ponies' drawing the coach.

The show reached a very high standard indeed and a great deal of hard work had obviously been put into it; although the stage was not very large, the cast of twenty-odd moved with absolute precision and never seemed to put a foot wrong or get in each other's way. The costumes, too, were absolutely magnificent, the Court Ladies' elaborate gowns even being topped with the correct tall wigs. When Cathy and the other three girls who represented the ponies appeared, they were dressed in the style of the famous Bluebell Girls, with satin leotards, fishnet tights, jewelled garters, ostrich plumes, the lot! We were so pleased that Cathy had lost her initial puppy-fat and now had a trim figure; we felt very proud of her in her elegant outfit and only wished we had brought a camera with us.

I felt that it was a great pity such an excellent show could not have had a longer run, so that members of the general public might have been admitted. It would, I am sure, have done a great deal of good and gone a long way towards counteracting the strange ideas that many people have about the mentally handicapped.

Shortly after this, excerpts were shown on TV of a similar production from a Centre elsewhere in the country. The reaction of the public was overwhelming and heart-warming; it really opened the eyes of many who saw the programme. Unfortunately, it was not very well advertised and was transmitted at a time of day when viewing figures usually slump. Unlike so many other things on television, it has never been repeated!

The *Cinderella* production whetted my appetite and I found myself planning how I could launch a drama group for the mentally handicapped. It was some time before this ambition was fulfilled, indeed it took the formation of the 'Thursday Club' to provide a suitable place for rehearsals.

This club — which was the brainchild of two or three parents — is a highly successful venture and has matured with the

years. Held in the local Community Centre, it caters for
mentally handicapped young people from the age of about
fourteen upwards.

It began with a handful of youngsters whom we brought in by
car, but now we have a membership of nearly a hundred, and
we use three minibuses, beside family cars; there are also those
who travel in by public transport or on foot. Besides the usual
youth club activities, such as pool, snooker, darts, table tennis
and dancing, we have an arts and crafts room, a cookery corner,
reading and writing classes and a coffee bar with comfortable
nooks for those who want simply to sit and chat. We also run
bingo sessions, a raffle or tombola and other varied events
which help to raise money for equipment and to pay for the
parties at Easter and Christmas. Every summer a beach barbecue is organised — a lot of fun with dancing on the sand,
singing and the consumption of quantities of hot dogs and coke.
The bonfire, which is lit down by the water, is carefully tended
by the husbands of the regular helpers, assisted by some of the
fathers — for parents are invited on this particular occasion.

Our latest activity is a drama class, which started in a small
way with four or five interested youngsters and took off from
there. Our would-be actors had mostly been involved before in
shows at the School and Centres, but they had always mimed
their parts to a spoken or taped commentary. We have gradually trained them to speak their own lines and hope to surprise
everyone some day by putting on a really spectacular show!
They have already graduated from short poems and sketches to
a Nativity play in five scenes. Our current production — our
most ambitious yet — is a full-length pantomime based on the
story of 'The Twelve Dancing Princesses'.

I find it extremely rewarding to work with mentally handicapped young people. A great deal of pleasure may be had, too,
from taking them out for the day; their enjoyment is so transparent, their wants so few. Added to this, they are usually far
better behaved than the average, run-of-the-mill coach party
and will wait patiently in orderly queues for the toilet, the
cafeteria or the odd fairground ride.

We have toured beautiful gardens in the pouring rain, safari parks in hermetically-sealed minibuses in blazing heat and beauty spots in a near-blizzard, but it never seemed to matter. We were always blessed with happy smiles — even chuckles at the worst bits — and the organisers came in for lots of grateful hugs and kisses at the end of the day.

*   *   *

Cathy had settled in well at Maybrook, when her twenty-first birthday arrived; the celebrations for this must surely have been the longest-running ever.

To begin with, we were on holiday in the Isle of Wight when the actual day came. A friend who was staying in the same hotel let the secret slip out and, on the morning of the great day, Cathy came in to breakfast to a table loaded with parcels and birthday cards. Every guest staying there had contributed something and I was greatly touched by their kindness. To crown everything, the friendly proprietors had baked her a special birthday cake and supplied a bottle of wine.

In the evening we had tickets for a play at nearby Sandown. Again our friend — who had booked the seats — had mentioned to the lady in the box office that it was a special birthday treat for a Down's girl who would be 21 on that day.

We arrived at the theatre early to find a veritable reception committee awaiting us in the foyer. The manager, producer, usherettes and any staff available were all standing in line ready to offer their congratulations; what was more, we were invited to visit backstage both before and after the show.

Eventually we were shown into the best seats in the house and presented with a free programme. We thoroughly enjoyed the show and, at the end, were invited into the bar where all the cast arrived, and then it was champagne all round!

Cathy was lifted on to a convenient table and everyone joined in with 'Happy Birthday to You!'. The nicest part about it was that the stars appearing in the show were all known to her from TV. A member of the *Coronation Street* cast, Hal Dyer from

Rent-a-Ghost and Janet Fielding from *Dr Who* all presented her afterwards with signed photographs; Cathy sailed back to the hotel with stars in her eyes!

The following day we arrived home after a long and arduous journey, occasioned by an inconvenient train strike. Piles of cards and presents were awaiting her from the family and all our friends. Next day we celebrated at a family luncheon-party and a few days later we had a barbecue and beach-picnic for all her handicapped friends. By that time the celebrations had lasted for six days! The most elongated twenty-first birthday I have ever heard of!

As I have said before, we have always tried to choose birthday and Christmas presents for Cathy that would not only give pleasure but also provide a certain amount of constructional or creative training.

Large picture-bricks and gaily-coloured 'build-ups', modelling clay, paints and pattern-makers have all added to her skills, and of course books of all kinds have always been top of the popularity list.

As she grew older, we tried to think of presents that would be more adult in concept and less like toys. A junior typewriter has been immensely popular (just like Mum's!), as was a glockenspiel and a beginner's guitar (just like my brother's!). The latter was put to very good use and she would sing along happily for hours, while strumming away at whatever 'chords' her fingers happened to light upon — excruciating for the rest of the family, who are all music-lovers, but Cathy was thoroughly entranced by her own accompaniment. We decided to grit our teeth and try to bear it! Fortunately she soon accepted the idea that hobbies such as this are much better practised in one's own room, which was a great relief to everyone!

To our surprise, however, she soon learned to pick out tunes on the glockenspiel by following the numbers written on the notes. We decided that, if she could do this, it was worth spending some time in teaching her that the *real* names of the notes were not '1, 2, 3 . . .' but 'A, B, C . . .'. Once she had mastered this fact, I bought a loose-leaf folder and made her her very own book of music, containing all her favourite songs and hymns. We still add new pages to this from time to time.

The other present that made quite a change in her life was a snooker table.

As soon as *Pot Black* was launched on TV, Cathy became an avid follower of snooker. I knew that she and several of her friends usually spent a while at the tables while at Thursday Club, but had never actually watched one of their games. I assumed that they enjoyed simply potting the different coloured balls and sending them into the pockets in whatever haphazard order happened to suit their fancy.

One evening at the club, Don beckoned me over to join him at the snooker table and indicated wordlessly that I should watch the game in progress. To my astonishment, Cathy and Stephen were playing a serious match, observing all the rules and even scoring correctly as they went along.

As soon as we realised that they were capable of doing this, we encouraged as many club members as possible to 'have a go'.

Quite soon afterwards, Chris supplied Cathy with a table-top model and she was able to practise at home as often as she liked, her game improving immediately. Although she does not play daily, as she did in the early days, she is still quite an addict and certainly loves to watch all the matches on TV. She is a great fan of all the champions, but her first favourite is definitely Steve Davis. She declares with great conviction that one day she intends to play against him — although I don't think she has any real hope of winning!

*　　*　　*

One of the most difficult things to teach a person with mental handicap is the danger of trusting strangers, and I really believe that this was one of my hardest tasks, so far as Cathy was concerned.

Like most Down's girls, she had such a friendly, affectionate nature; she had only to encounter the same traveller each day on the bus for that person to become her 'friend'.

It took quite a while to get her to accept that there were people in the world who might cause her harm and that even a familiar face was no sure passport to that person's integrity.

This awareness of danger, of course, is just as difficult a lesson to teach any of one's children. To protect the child without destroying its trust in others is a complicated business. These days, unfortunately, even blood relationship is no guarantee, and in reported cases of child molestation the percentage of incidents involving close relations and personal friends is frighteningly high.

My warnings must have been accepted finally, however, since the father of one of the other girls at Maybrook reported back to me that he had seen Cathy waiting at the bus stop one very wet day and offered her a ride home by car. She had refused politely, saying that she was not allowed to accept lifts and in any case preferred to travel by bus. Her refusal was made with a disarming smile and no one with good intentions could possibly have taken offence, her would-be driver told me; he added that he hoped his own daughter would be sensible enough to reply in the same way, if the occasion arose.

Sex instruction generally is difficult to convey to mentally handicapped persons. I found some of the television programmes for schools were very helpful, as they were couched in simple language intended for younger children, but were still quite explicit.

Cathy and I watched them together and I was able to answer her questions as they occurred to her. At the end of one such programme, which culminated in a film of the actual birth of a baby, she turned to me, her eyes shining, and said: 'Isn't it all wonderful?'

Chapter 9

When Marilyn — Leader of our Handicapped Rangers' Company — came to me in the Spring of 1981 and suggested that Cathy might like to work for a Duke of Edinburgh's Bronze Award, I looked at her blankly for a moment, since it was some years since I had had any involvement with the scheme.

It was first brought to my notice when Cathy was about thirteen years old. At one of our MENCAP Executive meetings, an item on the agenda announced that mentally handicapped young people were now being encouraged to compete in the Duke of Edinburgh's Award Scheme.

We considered this to be a tremendous breakthrough and assumed that, naturally, certain concessions would be made to allow for their handicap. On looking back, I realise that we were all a bit 'airy-fairy' about the whole thing, but certainly it seemed to be an interesting idea.

Cathy was too young at that time to participate and, of course, we did not in any case visualise a Down's child being able to take part. Some of the older boys and girls who were only slightly retarded were considered to be suitable, and classes were promptly arranged to cover various activities in which they could be given some basic training.

I was not actively involved on the teaching side, since I was certainly no expert on the subject of dressmaking, metalwork, swimming, sailing or any of the other skills that were being considered. I could have been classed as more of an interested onlooker and I thought it a great pity when numbers attending the courses began to dwindle and enthusiasm started to flag. Finally the whole plan seemed to disintegrate and — so far as out local youngsters were concerned — no more was heard of the Duke of Edinburgh's Awards.

In 1980, however, the scheme was totally revised and given a bit of a face-lift. Physically and mentally handicapped young people were again encouraged to take part and this was when Marilyn's interest was aroused; after a good deal of thought she came to the conclusion that Cathy might well be considered a suitable candidate.

We were naturally all in favour of her having a go. Even if she did not stay the course, she would probably find it interesting to travel at least part of the way. *En route*, she would certainly learn some new skills, and her horizons would inevitably be broadened.

Marilyn sent for the necessary handbooks and forms and we pored over them together. There were three Awards: Bronze, Silver and Gold, with a minimum starting age for each, the maximum age for completion being 25 years. Projects to be followed fell into four main sections: Service, Physical Recreation, Skills and Expeditions.

As far as the first category was concerned, the choice was easy. Cathy was already proving herself useful in the field of money-raising and working for charities. It meant simply widening the area in which she worked and teaching her how to keep a proper log of the time she had spent doing so. The requirement at Bronze level was for at least 60 hours of some sort of Community Service, spread over a year. Since most of the events at which she helped lasted for several hours at a time, this did not seem a difficult target to achieve.

Physical Recreation listed participation, improvement of performance and general progress as the main requirements. Our first choice was horse-riding, which was at that time her favourite sporting activity, and the only one in which she regularly took part; but we had to consider the 'improvement of performance' section. She had already advanced considerably, but at a riding school for the disabled, it was obvious that she would not be able to tackle the more difficult feats — such as jumping, for instance — and in any case, she had probably nearly reached her full potential.

Swimming seemed to be the obvious alternative. She had

enjoyed her sessions in the Lancaster School pool, conquered her early fear of water and, with the aid of arm-trainers, was beginning to master the correct basic strokes. She could probably improve on that level of performance and, even if she never reached the required standard for the Award, at least she would possibly learn to swim in the process — surely an essential thing for anyone who lived at the seaside or spent much time in the water.

The third category — Skills — was not so easy to pin down, though the choice was wide: from motor cycle maintenance through sculpture to astronomy!

We considered some of the activities that the handbook suggested. She had already dabbled in story-writing and acting — but it was doubtful that she would be able to study either to the high standard required; although she enjoyed drawing and painting, she was certainly no gifted artist; I had taught her to knit but she would probably not be able to master complicated patterns. Knitting, however, seemed to be the most likely choice from those offered and we decided to bear that in mind.

The final category of the Award Scheme was obviously going to be the most difficult one to tackle. It entailed an expedition or exploration which the candidate must plan and carry out more or less 'under his own steam'. We agreed that Cathy would probably never be able to achieve this particular part of the programme, so it should be left until the last and, if she never attempted it, it did not really matter. The whole purpose of the Duke of Edinburgh's Award Scheme was to encourage youngsters to 'expand' — to add new facets to their lives and to achieve their true potential. Since this had always been our aim with Cathy, it seemed a very good idea to let her take part.

After much discussion and thought we set the wheels in motion — having substituted needlework for knitting — and Cathy plunged in with great enthusiasm. Her programme had barely been launched when Marilyn rang me and suggested another consultation. When at last we managed to find the time to get together, she completely staggered me by suggesting that Cathy should skip the Bronze Award and set her sights higher.

'You mean the Silver?' I could not help sounding doubtful. I had always believed in the advisability of aiming high, but this seemed to me to be getting a little too ambitious.

'No.' Marilyn regarded me steadily and hesitated for only a moment or two. 'I mean the Gold.'

'You're crazy!' was my first reaction. No mentally handicapped person had at that time attempted the Gold Award. A few had embarked on the Bronze, but even they had not been Down's children.

'It would be marvellous if she could get it,' Marilyn pursued. 'Think what it would do for her — and for all the others. Wouldn't it be a tremendous step forward?'

I agreed that this was possibly the case. All the same, the idea seemed quite outrageous. She had already reached heights of prowess beyond our wildest dreams, but to believe that she could ever . . .

'It would have helped you, wouldn't it?' Marilyn was pointing out. 'When she was small — when you were being told constantly that Down's children couldn't do anything — supposing you'd heard about one of the older ones tackling something like that.'

She was right, of course. And as we talked it over I could see the other side of the argument. Cathy was now almost twenty, and it would take her possibly three years to achieve the Bronze Award; if she then went on to take the Silver, she would be too old to make an attempt for the Gold, and what a pity it would be if we found that by the time she was twenty-five she could actually have managed to reach the required level.

Why not, as Marilyn suggested, let her have a stab at it? The requirements were the same, it was just that the standard achieved had to be higher, the hours longer. If we found she wasn't going to make it, then we could always drop our sights and aim for the Bronze again. Everything really depended on Cathy herself. No way must she be badgered or chivvied along. If the whole business became a worry rather than a pleasure, then we would opt out of it; but the more we thought about it, the more sensible it seemed to strike out for the Gold . . .

We set out on this new and venturesome path rather tentatively and — on my part at any rate — with a few misgivings. As I have said previously, she was already quite involved in fund-raising activities. From the moment we began to work for MENCAP, we were caught up in a round-the-year cycle of fêtes, bazaars, jumble sales and other money-raising ventures. As soon as she was old enough to do so, Cathy had taken a great interest in the proceedings and always begged to be allowed to help. From the small start of putting the customer's money in the box provided, or holding out a container full of tombola tickets, she had finally graduated to having her own stall.

Michael had made her a 'spinning wheel' with different coloured sections representing different grades of prizes to be won, for which the customers had to spin an arrow to try to win the prize of their choice. He later constructed a more sophisticated version of this in the shape of a grandfather clock. The minute hand moved round the face, to stop eventually at a particular time on the clock. Behind each number on the dial was a little door which the customer opened, to find the mystery prize behind it.

Children particularly loved this side-show, and Cathy always had a large crowd round her 'Dickery Dock Clock' and was kept very busy taking money, giving instructions and keeping the little boxes behind the doors filled. Apart from the pleasure it gave her, it was an excellent training ground.

By keeping the price on all her stalls at 10p a go, we were able to ensure that she could manage the money side of the business on her own. She soon learned to give the correct change for a proffered 50p or £1 note. Constant practice helped her later to work out more complicated transactions!

As well as helping our own Society, she enjoyed setting up her stall at other events. There were church fêtes and bazaars, of course, to say nothing of events for the Guide and Scout companies in which she and Michael were involved. We also went along to help a friend with a garden party at a local home for the blind. This led to other visits; Cathy found a natural affinity with blind people and was able to include them in her Community Service.

She soon learned how to keep an accurate log of the time she had spent on these activities, how much money she had raised and what the work actually involved. There were other facets, too, to this form of service. She was greatly interested in *See, Hear* and other television programmes made specially for the deaf; it was her own idea to learn the deaf and dumb alphabet and some of the sign language, so that she could communicate with anyone with this disability. Surprisingly, she picked it up very quickly and has retained the knowledge; but there is no doubt in my own mind that Down's children have great visual ability and find this kind of learning much easier to assimilate.

In this particular project she was expected to know a little about the various charities for which she was working. This entailed collecting leaflets and pamphlets and learning about the local facilities provided for the elderly and persons with disabilities. She was expected to carry out her Community Service for at least eighteen months, but of course she continued working for charities for a good deal longer than this – and, needless to say, is still doing so.

When it came to her Physical Recreation, she took to the water like the proverbial duck and, in her enthusiasm, was soon able to swim unassisted.

Maybrook now virtually took over this section of the Award and undertook to see her through it; I am most grateful for their interest and dedication, for it took a lot of the work off our shoulders. At about this time the Maybrook instructors had decided to engage the services of a professional swimming coach to help with the groups of trainees who went weekly to the local baths. Once launched on this training programme, Cathy's performance immediately improved, and very soon afterwards she was able to take her first test; she came home proudly displaying a badge bearing the words 'Water Skills Grade I'.

The next stage, after a series of exercises to get her used to swimming with her face under water, was to try to practise covering longer distances. In a surprisingly short while she had achieved the badge for 10 metres length, then another for 25 metres, quickly followed by 50 metres. After this there was no stopping her!

This part of the Award was satisfactorily completed, although again she was expected to continue with her training for a reasonable amount of time. Obviously, though, swimming is another activity that Cathy thoroughly enjoys and presumably she intends to go on with it and perhaps to become even more proficient as a swimmer.

This, of course, is what the Duke of Edinburgh's Scheme is all about. Prince Philip's main concern has been that young people, having reached their target, should continue to participate in their chosen sports, hobbies or services.

At first consideration, the requirements for the needlework section seemed numerous and quite difficult for a virtual beginner. Having followed a course of lessons for at least a year, she must at the end of that time have completed at least one garment. The finished article should demonstrate ability to carry out a number of skills, including: setting-in a zip, button-holes, gathers, darts, a collar and cuffs, hand-finishing and also proficient use of a sewing-machine.

After scouring a number of shops, I was quite unable to find the pattern of a garment that included all of those things. So we compromised in the end by deciding to make two articles: trousers and a separate top.

Initially, of course, Cathy had to practise on odd pieces of material and all these early attempts had to be kept for the final adjudication, so that her general progress could be observed. My workbox soon began to look like something out of a tailor's nightmare, so we had to find other accommodation for the various weird and wonderful 'first tries'.

She soon began to get the hang of the thing, however, and we were able to find a small second-hand sewing-machine on which she could practise at home, since her needlework sessions actually took place at our Thursday Club. Gail, her teacher and guide, showed endless patience and with gentle persuasion soon ironed out any problems.

It took Cathy about eighteen months in all to complete her project. The resulting garments, at the end of all this, reached a standard beyond our wildest hopes and have been included in so many exhibitions and displays that, as yet, she has not been able to get around to wearing them!

For the final part of this section, she was asked to design a book of clothes which would suit her own particular figure. As she was not very good at drawing, she began by tracing pictures from the magazines and adapting them slightly to her own taste. Eventually, however, after a long search, I tracked down something that would help her.

Called a 'Fashion Wheel', it was an ingenious device in which templates of various types of skirts, bodices, sleeves, etc., were used to create original designs. The permutations between the pieces were enormous and as the 'wheels' involved were quite simple to use, she was soon able to complete the rest of her project.

Incidentally, I would highly recommend this fascinating fashion-maker for the use of any mentally handicapped child with artistic leanings. Manufactured by Milton Bradley Ltd., under the name of 'MB Toys', and apparently made in West Germany, it is quite hard to find in the shops but well worth looking for.

Cathy had already achieved a residential qualification, which is one of the first requirements for entering the Award Scheme. The candidate was expected to spend a week in some place such as a camp or youth hostel and, during the stay, he or she would be assessed for general behaviour, politeness, willingness to help, personal appearance and so on. Cathy's testing time took place while she was camping with the Handicapped Guides and Rangers. Unknown to her, she was being carefully watched for the duration of the holiday and she received a very good report from her Assessor, who marked her highly in every category.

*   *   *

Most of the hurdles had now been passed, but at long last we came to the really difficult part. The Expedition or Exploration category had been something we had put to the back of our minds, since it seemed unlikely that she would ever be able to reach the extremely high standard required.

It meant going far away from home, possibly into 'wild' country, learning to map-read and to plan a journey which included many miles of walking and possibly climbing or pioneering. At the end of it all, a log must be produced which would have to be well-written and include photographs and any specimens collected on the way.

The only thing to do was to let her undertake the three 'dummy runs' which were required of her before she tackled the final journey. On three different occasions, therefore, she went youth hostelling with a group of other Maybrook trainees — under supervision, naturally. This prepared her for the routine followed when staying in a hostel and showed her how the next day's journey could be planned in advance; it also gave her practice in writing her log, for on each occasion she made notes of all that she had done and what kind of meals she had eaten.

In the meantime, Marilyn was trying to find a suitable location for the final test. Our first idea — of linking her up with a party of other girls taking the Award — never came to fruition and we had to accept finally that she would have to 'go it alone'. We also met up with the kind of prejudice which is shown so often by members of the general public. Several times Marilyn arranged for her to visit certain locations for exploration purposes; permission would be freely given, but it was as quickly withdrawn once the information was passed on that it was a mentally handicapped girl who would be working on the project.

The next step, therefore, was to find a party of three other people who would be willing to go with her. Her friend Avril — also a Down's girl — was very anxious to accompany her and the group was completed by two sisters, Jo and Sarah Hurley, from a local Venture Scout Unit. They, of course, were not handicapped and I can never thank them enough for their sensible attitude to Cathy. Without interfering in any way or diminishing her leadership, they were immensely supportive and ready to do anything they were asked.

Being intelligent girls and very active physically, it must have been somewhat frustrating, to say the least, to have to travel at the pace of the other two girls; but they never lost patience or tried to hurry them in any way.

The locality chosen for the Exploration was Epping Forest. The youth hostel where they would be staying was at High Beech, within visiting distance of Waltham Abbey and other historic buildings which could be used on the project.

Cathy herself had to write the letters to the hostel, making the booking, and to the Conservation Centre and other places of interest they hoped to visit.

She had already undertaken a certain amount of training in first aid, map-reading and the country code. It was necessary, too, to practise taking photographs — of which she would need a large number for illustrating her log — and to learn to use a flower-press, so that specimens could be preserved and brought back with her.

Added to this, she had to be responsible for feeding her party. This meant working out suitable menus which — as well as being considered well-balanced by her Assessor — would also consist of ingredients that were easily obtainable and not too complicated to cook.

By the time the girls were ready to set off, she had made copious notes about each day's itinerary, the routes to be taken and which places they must make a point of visiting.

She had already planned the journeys to and from High Beach. This meant finding out the times of trains and buses and where the connections must be made. She would be responsible for the safe conduct of her party and, for their part, while carrying out her instructions, they must at the same time not make suggestions or try to influence her in any way.

The day before they left, we all met up for the last time: Marilyn, myself, Cathy, the other girls and the Assessor who had to examine all the plans and preparations she had made and then decide whether or not she had completed this part of the programme to his satisfaction.

He spent a long time talking to her and firing questions at intervals, in order to make sure that everything was quite clear in her mind; she answered all of them correctly and was able to give him all the relevant information, even to the colour of the bus she hoped to catch at the start of the journey! He told me later that he had purposely been quite tough on her, to ensure that no one afterwards could say she had been allowed any concessions because of her handicap.

In fact, everything that she did to attain the award was carried out in exactly the same way any participant would follow. This met with our full approval; to have lowered the required standards — even if that had been possible — would have defeated the whole purpose of the exercise.

On the great day, the four girls met at our house early in the morning. As I watched them set off, heavy knapsacks on their backs and wearing the sensible shoes they would need for the long walk at the end of the journey, I was suddenly filled with a sickening sense of dismay.

What kind of mother was I to let my handicapped daughter set out on such a very difficult exercise? In trying to bring out the best in her and let her realise her full potential, had I finally gone too far and set her an impossible task? Perhaps I *was* just as irresponsible as so many people had suggested over the years.

I went slowly into the house and spent a day plunged in deep depression, with occasional flashes of intense anxiety in case anything had gone wrong. Late in the afternoon I answered the 'phone and found that my caller was Cathy herself. She sounded so happy and was obviously extremely proud of having arrived safely at the hostel without any hitches. They had taken two buses, a train and walked the last part of the way, paying a visit to Waltham Abbey *en route*. In the background I could hear the laughing voices of the other girls, and they all seemed to be enjoying themselves immensely.

My feeling of relief is quite impossible to describe. I knew at that moment that everything was going to be all right.

The girls spent five days away from home. They visited many places of interest and explored the forests, examining the flora and fauna and bringing back some interesting specimens. Cathy took two complete films of photographs and most of them turned out very well indeed.

Each day's exploits were written up in note-books and they shared the chores of cooking the evening meal, making up packed lunches for the following day and helping to keep the youth hostel clean and tidy. Altogether they covered a considerable number of miles.

The journey home — taking a different route this time — was completed without disaster and it was easy to see that, although tired and somewhat travel-worn, they had all enjoyed themselves very much. For the other three, the Exploration was over, but on Cathy's part quite a lot of work had still to be done. She would have to write up the log of their activities and illustrate it with the photographs and specimens she had brought back with her.

After a few days' rest, she embarked on this long and arduous task. What would have taken most people two or three evenings to complete, absorbed her for several weeks. As usual, she did not want to stop work until the whole thing was finished. I had to be very firm with her to ensure she did not overdo things, but she stuck to her task doggedly and finally managed to reach the end.

We were told later that it was one of the best logs the examiners had received. It was certainly something of which she could afford to be proud. Cathy is a very neat writer and obviously enjoyed laying out the pages tidily. The only thing we had to help her with was — as usual! — her spelling.

By the end of July her work had been handed in and she had met another Assessor and been questioned at length by him. He gave us a very encouraging report and said that he had no hesitation in passing her for that particular part of the Award.

Next her record book, which contained the various Assessors' reports, had to be sent in with the log and anything else of relevance. Then began a long and wearisome wait. It was not until just before Christmas that we learned she had gained her Award and would be presented with her Gold Badge at County Hall, Chelmsford, in January. What a really exciting Christmas present to give us!

*   *   *

We had been warned that, once the news of her success was announced, 'all hell could break loose'! How very true that was. Splashed all over the local papers — who gave us really splendid coverage — the story was soon picked up by the national dailies and we were besieged by reporters and photographers, all anxious to have an exclusive interview. We spoke to all of them, although, needless to say, some of the stories never appeared at all and others were reduced to a small paragraph in an obscure corner. Two very good articles appeared in the *Daily Mail* and the *Daily Telegraph*, however, and later we were interviewed by *Woman's Own*, who produced a 'spread' with pictures, as part of their Down's children series.

On the day when we were due to travel to Chelmsford where Cathy would receive her gold brooch at County Hall, I was contacted by Thames Television, who wanted to come down and film her for possible inclusion in that evening's news bulletin.

Since they could not give me an exact time of arrival, I suggested that they might prefer to meet Cathy at Maybrook, where she worked, rather than at home. In this way she would not have to ask for a day's leave and they might, in any case, like to film her in her work surroundings.

What a blessing it was that I had that idea! We would never have coped in an ordinary house. By 9.00 a.m. a camera and sound crew, plus reporters, had arrived from Thames TV, to be followed at short intervals by similar units from ITN, Anglia and the BBC *London Plus* programme!

Maybrook was turned upside down and inside out as lights, cables and cameras materialised everywhere, soon to be joined by a team from BBC Radio. Fortunately Maybrook's Manager and staff were most co-operative and took everything in their stride and, of course, the trainees were absolutely delighted by all that was going on!

From soon after 9.00 o'clock until about 3.30 p.m., I dashed from room to room giving interviews and posing for camera shots. As the time went on and the lights seemed to grow hotter and hotter and hotter, I felt myself becoming more and more dishevelled, but there was no time for running repairs! Cathy was called in to join me once or twice for a joint interview, but for most of the day she continued with her job of preparing and serving the lunches, setting tables, washing-up and so on, and not turning a hair at being filmed in the process. The TV people were all much amused at her coolness and ability to carry on as normal, despite all that was happening around her; but it was, of course, this sense of purpose and dedication that had already helped her, against all odds, to reach Gold Award standard.

Once or twice she raised a smile, especially when she looked back over her shoulder with a wicked grin and told the camera man to be careful or he'd get his camera all steamed up. Later, while I was explaining to the interviewer that when Cathy was small I had been told that she wouldn't be able to do very much at all, she turned to me and said, 'Yes, but I can do quite a lot now, can't I, Mum?' Both incidents were televised.

It was a most interesting — and chaotic — day. For my own part, the worst thing of all was not having anything to eat or drink for several hours. Lucy, in charge of the kitchens at Maybrook, had put aside some lunch for me, and tea and coffee appeared as if by magic at half-hourly intervals throughout the day, for the benefit of the TV and Radio crews; but every time I gratefully reached out for a cup I was whisked away to another part of the Centre for some more filming. I had great fellow-feeling for the tormented Tantalus with his everlasting thirst!

Eventually we were free to go, but we had barely an hour in which to return home and have a hasty wash-and-brush-up before setting out for County Hall, Chelmsford, where Cathy was to be presented with her Gold Brooch by Robert Heron, Director of the Duke of Edinburgh's Award Scheme.

It was a bitterly cold evening and beginning to snow. Christopher drove us there and we had a hilarious journey as out daughter-in-law, Mary, gave Cathy a blow-wave as we drove alone, in an attempt to repair the ravages of the day's filming.

We managed to find the hall eventually and, accompanied by Marilyn and Don and the other members of the family, I was lucky enough to have a seat in the front row, from where we were able to get a good view of the proceedings. The ceremony went off beautifully, with thirty youngsters from all over Essex receiving their Awards. All had been won during the past year.

When the presentations were being made, a halt was called just before Cathy made her appearance. The Chairman announced that, in twenty years of Award Ceremonies, no name had ever been singled out for a special mention. However, he felt that on this occasion an exception had to be made. He gave a brief summary of all that Cathy had achieved, adding: 'It really is beyond me or anyone else to put into words the amount of effort she has had to put in.' The applause that followed was deafening, cameras all round us flashed and, on our part, we found it a moment charged with emotion. So many years of hoping, believing and tremendous hard work on Cathy's part had culminated in this peak of her triumph.

We left the hall, somewhat bemused, and met Cathy in the foyer. Having been deprived of sustenance for most of the day I, for one, was delighted to see the mouth-watering buffet that had been set out for the candidates and their families. However, my pleasure was short-lived! Before we could manage more than a nibble, we were besieged by reporters and photographers who all wanted separate interviews, of course.

When, eventually, we arrived home, we were just in time to hear the 'phone ringing. It was TVS on the line asking for our permission to use excerpts that they had 'borrowed' from the film that Anglia had made; these were to be transmitted on their ten o'clock news bulletin, which was about to go on the air.

I readily gave permission and hastily switched on the TV set. This time we were able to view ourselves on the news programme that followed, having missed our other appearances throughout the day. Altogether Cathy's story was featured on four different channels at 1.00 o'clock, 5.00, 6.00, 7.00, 8.00, 9.00 and 10.00 p.m. We also broadcast on Radio 1, Radio 3, Radio 4 and 'made' the World News on the following morning.

For days afterwards, our 'phone barely stopped ringing as old and new friends contacted us — and then the cards and letters began to arrive and continued to do so for a long while afterwards. Many of the telephone calls and letters came from complete strangers; receiving these was undoubtedly a most moving and heart-warming experience.

The large number of letters we had from other parents of handicapped children — most of them unknown to us — made me realise that, apart from anything else, at least we had managed to convey the message that the Down's Children's Association had been so anxious for us to hammer home: namely, that these children, with the right amount of encouragement and careful training, can reach heights not so far dreamt of. I was left with a feeling of wonderment that what we had set out to do for Cathy's sake alone, was now probably going to benefit many other children, too.

Having weathered this first spate of publicity, we knew that public interest would probably be aroused once more when Cathy later visited St James's Palace to meet Prince Philip. Until then, I knew that life would probably be quite hectic, since invitations for personal appearances had begun to pour in and I was already being asked to fulfil more speaking engagements than I could possibly manage. What else the future would hold we did not know, but whatever emerged I felt that I was beyond being surprised . . .

Chapter 10

If I have a message to share at all, it is this:

Never, *never* accept the statement that your child is 'ineducable'. Even the most handicapped person can be taught to do *something*.

You will need strong determination and a great deal of courage, for many of the so-called 'experts' will laugh at your hopes and assure you cynically that it is much better to accept your child's shortcomings right from the start and learn to live with them.

I, personally, was offered nothing but discouragement all the way along the line, and if I had been prepared to accept the verbal label that was attached to our daughter, she would never have learned to do anything. Well, perhaps she would have acquired some basic skills, for the kindness and patience of the Staff at Lancaster School and Maybrook Centre would have seen to that. But however good the level of teaching and however dedicated the teacher, success cannot really be guaranteed without steady backing from home; for even with the best of intentions, staff at Training Centres cannot give as much individual attention as they would like to each child.

If my mother had not fought for me every inch of the way, I would never have walked again. If we, as a family, had not set out to ensure that Cathy was given every chance to attain her true potential, she would not be the happy, vital, totally fulfilled young woman that she is now.

To achieve the Duke of Edinburgh's Gold Award — and to be the first Down's child to do so — was an extra bonus that was added on the way. We did not set out to make her famous in her own little world; it was just something that evolved from the rest of the training.

Apart from the full life she leads and all the pleasure she gets from taking part in so many varied activities, she herself has added warmth to the lives of many other people, radiating love and friendship to those about her.

Our other children have, I am sure, also learned something in the process: patience, to be really caring and to have sympathy for the elderly, the under-privileged and the handicapped.

In a recent television programme, the elder sister of a teen-aged Down's boy insisted that such children should be allowed to die at birth. 'After all,' she announced carelessly, but with absolute conviction, 'you can't call them *people*, can you?'

I found this to be not so much shocking as very, very sad. From his brief appearance on the programme, her brother appeared to be what is often termed 'high-grade'; he had been institutionalised at an early age and allowed to make only brief visits home, and on these occasions his sister obviously tried her best to keep out of his way.

What a pity she had not been given the chance to get to know and learn to love him; she might not then have matured into the rather cynical, uncaring twenty-year-old that she appeared to be.

Of course there are times when a mentally handicapped child is a good deal better off in care than in his or her own home. This is also true of many 'normal' children, and each case must be considered on its own merit. But I am assuming that if you are a parent of a Down's boy or girl and are reading this book, then you are sufficiently interested in your child's future to want to do your damnedest to ensure the best for him or her.

Certainly, there will be heartaches and there will be disappointments and occasionally —when you are very tired, for instance — you will wonder why you should bother at all. But life generally is like that and we all feel the urge to opt out at times. Then, suddenly, will come the breakthrough and the joy of seeing your child suddenly acquire a new skill — and how rewarding the warm rush of happiness when you catch sight of the expression of wonder on his face. For there is no doubt about it: your sense of triumph will be trebled for the child himself.

Since finishing the first draft of this book, I have found myself wondering whether to write another chapter. For Cathy is beginning to add to the skills she has already mastered. Then I realised that, as long as she lives, there need be no real end to her story. Like any other interested adult, she can take up new hobbies and discard them at will. Because of her reading ability she can widen her scope and tackle a different kind of book; this, in turn, will often prompt her to try a new type of activity, and so it goes on . . .

I have been amused recently — I am beyond being surprised — when, on more than one occasion, she has been able to answer a question that has baffled contestants on *University Challenge* or *Mastermind* (two programmes she loves to watch.)

'How did you know that?' I asked her once and was told airily, 'Oh, I read it in one of my books.'

She does not remember everything she reads, of course, but obviously quite a lot of it *does* stick.

I look back sometimes on those early days, when I was told repeatedly that she was unlikely to learn very much, that it was better to accept the inevitable and not to aim too high, because it would bring only disappointment and heartache.

I meet many parents who have accepted this philosophy and learned to live with their child's handicap and to be grateful because he or she is not too difficult to handle. I am pleased for their sake that they are able to feel reasonably content. Then I look more closely at the child and sometimes it saddens me greatly to see so much potential wasted, so much initiative strangled at an early age.

At Thursday Club we try to teach some of these young people skills that they have never before learned and parents are usually astonished at the outcome. But for some it is too late; the pattern has already been set and that little spark of initiative has been extinguished. We still persevere with them, of course, but too often it is like fighting a losing battle. Nevertheless, it is worth the effort, for who can say how much is absorbed in the process?

I can remember one particular incident, concerning a boy who would probably be labelled by Society generally as 'a cabbage'. He suddenly came to life when a record of *The Sound of Music* was played to him. For one short minute, while Julie Andrews sang 'Doh-a-Deer', he rocked himself in time to the music and a glint of animation showed in his eyes. Then it was all over. He relapsed once more into his habitual apathy and I never knew him to respond again. I have wondered many times since exactly what went through his mind at that moment.

I could give many more examples: the boy who always wasted the entire evening running aimlessly round and round the clubroom — until we discovered he had a talent for painting; the young man who could not talk but was taught to play an excellent game of table tennis; the girl who used to retire into the remotest corner and remain there, yet ventured out finally and learned to cook.

Our team of dedicated workers pursue every avenue until some activity is found to suit each handicapped member. The display of Easter Bonnets this year — *everyone*, with help, made one to wear — had to be seen to be believed!

*   *   *

And now, what of the future? This is a question I am so often asked. There are many variations in the phrasing, but they really all mean the same thing:

'Don't you worry constantly about what will happen to her?'

'Can you bear to look ahead?'

'Isn't the thought of the future a terrible nightmare?'

'She has had so much love, but what will happen to her when you die?'

Some years ago I was asked to contribute to a certain publication and I wrote the following words:

One dark shadow looms. It is the thought that constantly haunts every parent of a mentally handicapped child — and a day never passes when I do not ask myself the chilling questions: 'What is to become of our daughter when we are no longer here? Who will house her, protect her and care for her needs? Where will she go . . . who will want her?

But that, as I say, was some years ago. I feel differently now. We have done our best to make her as independent as possible and taught her the kind of skills she will need to have in order to live outside the shelter of the family home.

As to where she will go . . . I have faith in God's infinite wisdom and I truly believe that the right niche will be found for her. Hopefully, this will come about while we are still here and able to see her comfortably installed. In this way it will be a gentle process, with visits to and from those at home, until she has settled happily into the new environment. At all costs, we should like to spare her the burden of living with aged and over-dependent parents, culminating in the shock of being suddenly bereaved and hastily thrust into some new way of life. I hope that we shall be unselfish enough to let her go when the right moment comes.

But whatever the future holds, I am quite sure she will be well looked after. We are lucky enough to have three other children and a very dear daughter-in-law and son-in-law, whom we know will always have Cathy's welfare at heart.

And, most important of all, there is the comforting thought of 'Someone up there' who, I am sure, has a special affection for this youngest child of ours. He must count her a prize to be valued. Why, otherwise, would He have lent her to us as a special blessing and filled her heart so full of joy and love?

I am very conscious of the privilege of having been asked to share in her life. So, I shall borrow a phrase from Cathy herself and say, with all humility:

Thanks, God!

Useful addresses

The Down's Children's Association
  4 Oxford Street, London W1N 9FL. Tel: 01–580 0511/2
  For helping parents and professionals with the care, treatment and training of children with Down's Syndrome.
The Makaton Vocabulary Development Project
  31 Firwood Drive, Camberley, Surrey, GU15 3QD.
  Makaton is a sign language that has been found to encourage the development of language in Down's children.
MENCAP (the Royal Society for Mentally Handicapped Children and Adults)
  123 Golden Lane, London EC1Y ORT. Tel: 01–253 9433
  For increasing public awareness and understanding of the problems of mentally handicapped people.
National Portage and Home Teaching Association
  R.J. Cameron, Winchester Portage Service, Silver Hill, Winchester SO23 8AF.
  A system of home education for young pre-school children who have special educational needs.
Play Matters (The Toy Libraries Association)
  Seabrook House, Wyllyotts Manor, Darkes Lane, Potters Bar, Herts. EN6 2HL.

Some helpful books

COPELAND, James, and HODGES, Jack (1973). *For the Love of Ann*, London: Arrow Books.

COTTON, Mike (1981). *Out of Doors with Handicapped People*, London: Souvenir Press.

COTTON, Mike (1983). *Outdoor Adventure for Handicapped People*, London: Souvenir Press.

CRAIG, Mary (1979). *Blessings*, London: Hodder & Stoughton.

CUNNINGHAM, Cliff (1982). *Down's Syndrome: An Introduction for Parents*, London: Souvenir Press.

CUNNINGHAM, Cliff, and SLOPER, Patricia (1978). *Helping Your Handicapped Baby*, London: Souvenir Press.

D'ARCY, Paula (1981). *Song for Sarah*, Tring, Herts.: Lion Publishing.

JEFFREE, Dorothy M., and CHESELDINE, Sally (1984). *Let's Join In*, London: Souvenir Press.

JEFFREE, Dorothy M., and McCONKEY, Roy (1976). *Let Me Speak*, London: Souvenir Press.

JEFFREE, Dorothy M., McCONKEY, Roy, and HEWSON, Simon (1985). *Let Me Play*, second edition, London: Souvenir Press.

JEFFREE, Dorothy M., and SKEFFINGTON, Margaret (1980). *Let Me Read*, London: Souvenir Press.

McCONKEY, Roy, and McCORMACK, Bob (1983). *Breaking Barriers: Educating People about Disability*, London: Souvenir Press.

PHILPS, Caroline (1984). *Elizabeth Joy: A Mother's Story*, Tring, Herts.: Lion Publishing.

SANCTUARY, Gerald (1984). *After I'm Gone: What Will Happen to My Handicapped Child?*, London: Souvenir Press.

SHENNAN, Victoria (1983). *A Home of Their Own*, London: Souvenir Press.

WEST, Morris (1981). *The Clowns of God*, London: Hodder & Stoughton.

WHELAN, Edward, and SPEAKE, Barbara (1981). *Getting to Work*, London: Souvenir Press.

WHELAN, Edward, and SPEAKE, Barbara (1979). *Learning to Cope*, London: Souvenir Press.

WILLIAMS, Paul, and SHOULTZ, Bonnie (1982). *We Can Speak for Ourselves: Self-advocacy by mentally handicapped people*, London: Souvenir Press.